WOW,
Your Mom Really Is
C R A Z Y

WOW,
Your Mom Really Is
C R A Z Y

A Complete Guide to Coping with Thyroid Disease:
Stress, Weight Loss Tips, and More

CAROL GRAY

iUniverse, Inc.
Bloomington

Wow, Your Mom Really Is Crazy
A Complete Guide to Coping with Thyroid Disease: Stress, Weight Loss Tips, and More

iUniverse books may be ordered through booksellers or by contacting:

iUniverse
1663 Liberty Drive
Bloomington, IN 47403
www.iuniverse.com
1-800-Authors (1-800-288-4677)

ISBN: 978-1-4759-5349-7 (sc)
ISBN: 978-1-4759-5351-0 (hc)
ISBN: 978-1-4759-5350-3 (ebk)

Library of Congress Control Number: 2012918915

Printed in the United States of America

iUniverse rev. date: 10/10/2012

Table of Contents

Introduction

It is estimated that fifty million Americans suffer from autoimmune diseases, such as rheumatoid arthritis, fibromyalgia, Crohn's disease, and lupus (aarda.org, 2011). Fifty million is roughly equivalent to the combined populations of California and Texas. Nearly twelve million Americans have a thyroid disease, such as Hashimoto's disease, Graves' disease, or cancer (Harvard, 2011). I have both a thyroid disease and an autoimmune disease. This book tells the story of my journey from sanity to psychosis to comfortably crazy.

Ten years ago my husband, son and I moved into an upper-middle-class neighborhood filled with stay-at-home moms, green lawns, mischievous children, and white-collar dads in their loosened ties. I was never really one to put on airs, but in *this* neighborhood, I tried to be more like the Joneses. Upgrading from an apartment to a tiny starter home and finally to our new place was essential. We had to keep moving into bigger dwellings because my son's toys were taking over; his stuffed animals alone could populate the jungles of Africa. As we continued to expand, our living space wasn't the only thing getting bigger: my physical and mental problems were also growing. Most of those who suffer from autoimmune diseases are usually sick an average of ten years with various ailments before they finally receive the correct diagnoses. I was no exception. I was turning into a *Looney Tunes* character but was keeping this behind closed doors, of course, because in suburbia, everyone is perfect . . . right? My neighbors had no idea that I wasn't. It was like sucking in my gut, so to speak, to the outside world—and then letting it all hang out with my husband and son. Lucky them.

So there I was in my big-girl house with my big-girl mortgage, trying to appear like just another suburbanite. My time was spent flowering, manicuring, hedging, trimming, and watering; yard work is truly a full-time job. A *perfectly* manicured lawn wasn't my thing, but I may have been trying to overcompensate for the imperfections that were brewing within. I was actually trying to hide behind the façade. Other pretentious residential activities included tossing the ball with the neighborhood kiddos (including the brats) at the appropriate time of day: a half hour before dinner or an hour after dinner. Waving and smiling those pearly whites at folks I most certainly could not pick out of a criminal lineup if my life depended on it. ("Oh, that's one of my *neighbors . . . ?* Really, are you sure, officer?")

It was a gorgeous day in the neighborhood—opulent sunshine with the perfect amount of wind. I had all the windows open so I could feel the warm breeze coming into my house. This was an ideal spring-cleaning day. The outside of my home was picture perfect, so now it was time to clean the inside. The front door was open, but we had a screen door to keep the bugs out.

While diligently dusting the furniture, I heard his little voice say, "Mommy, Mommy!"

"What, honey?"

"Can me and Zach get some ice cream from the ice-cream man?"

"I don't have any money, babe."

"I do, Mommy."

Of course you do. You always have money—more than me, I thought. I walked to his room to get his piggy bank, filled more with green than metal. While walking back to the screen door, I noticed both little boys were looking so enthusiastic. You could just see it in their eyes; they were visualizing the tasty ice-cream treats, which would later be a melting mess for me to clean up. In an instant I realized that playing a prank on them was an opportunity I could not pass up. Approaching the screen door, clutching the giant pink pig in my hands, I roared, "*Muuwaahhhhh!* You think you boys are getting some ice cream?"—gnashing my teeth, trying to do my best Peter Lorre impression—"No way! The money's all mine—all mine, I tell you! *Muwaaahhhh!*"

The eerie crinkling noise produced by my lemony Pledge-covered hands was perhaps a little too theatrical for someone else's child. My son was used to my behavior, but Zach's mouth dropped to the ground. Tyler stared at his mother with no interest. Both boys were just as cute as buttons. Even though there was a screen door between Zach and me, he still looked terrified. He looked at me with this perplexed, frightened gaze, and then he looked over at Tyler and said, "Wow, Tyler, you were right. Your mom *really is* crazy."

When Zach said this, I immediately started laughing hysterically. This little guy was afraid of his best friend's mommy? Then my laughter promptly shifted to panic. *Oh my God! Zach is seeing me act this way!* I thought. Suddenly, I caught a quick glimpse into my future; everyone knowing the real me was a scary notion. You see, the hard work and dedication that Zach's mom puts into her gossiping is unlike anything I have ever seen. My paranoia was valid—this time.

I firmly believe Zach's mom has a secret passageway behind her washer and dryer. This is where she clandestinely slips into her underground bunker to send out gossip via Morse code. This "news" is then distributed throughout the neighborhood and surrounding counties, and to the rest of the state, the country, and parts of Europe, all before sundown. This time the message would say the following: *There is a crazy woman living at 725 Meadow Lark Drive in Carmel, IN.* I would be outed. The jig was up.

Oh well, I thought to myself, *I might as well face the music*. My transition from laughter to panic soon gave way to relief. One of the best things about having a bum thyroid is that a massive emotional shift can happen in seconds. Little-known fact: when a dramatic actor in a movie instantaneously goes from laughing deliriously to crying, she is portraying someone with a thyroid disease. I'm sure of it.

After I was outed, my mental and physical condition began to rapidly deteriorate. I was becoming extremely sick and had no idea why. At the pinnacle of my illness, when I believed there was no way I could get any sicker, my diagnosis came. Consequently, my fake smiles ended; I stopped playing ball with the brats, and instead they received my snarls. My once-pristine yard started looking like the Addams Family dwelling.

Looking back on it all, I can see that it was silly to hide what I was going through. But when one is sick and has no idea what is wrong, this causes an enormous amount of fear. The worst possible diagnoses swirled secretly in my mind. Hoping and pretending it would all go away, I tried as best I could to act like I was well. Finally getting a diagnosis was a relief. I think this was because I finally had an answer. When you *know* you are sick and then you get confirmation, you can let out a big sigh of relief—and let it all hang out!

—

What you can expect from this book:

1. Cheesy movie and television references: I love movies and television. I had to turn off the TV to write this book, and it about killed me.
2. Grids, charts, and diagrams: Only thyroid sufferers will know why this is essential.
3. MacGraver tips: I used to be a loyal *MacGyver* viewer. I have created tips on how to cope with my thyroid disease, Graves' disease. My tips are called "MacGraver tips." Tee-hee—get it?
4. Humor
5. My thyroid insanity: Raw, uncut, and uncensored. I firmly believe that most mental health issues and related behaviors of a thyroid sufferer have not been fully documented and/ or recognized by the scientific and medical communities.
6. MacGraver tips from other autoimmune disease sufferers
7. Twelve steps for the thyroid sufferer (**Note:** The twelve-step process for addicts has a core spiritual foundation, yet its

founders and current organizers accept *all* who seek sobriety within this proven, widespread program. My twelve steps for the thyroid sufferer are nondiscriminatory as well; atheists are welcome to read. But, I want this book to be for all; therefore if you are an atheist, you may skip chapter 7(the spiritual chapter.)

Chapter 1

Stress, the Bad Kind

I want you to close your eyes and try to go back in time to remember a specific event in your life. Now, I know this is asking an awful lot of you, my thyroid-deficient friend. No one knows more than I do how difficult it is to conjure up memories. But I would venture to guess that the particular memory I am going to ask you to reflect on is probably still very strong because it relates to that spiteful, sinister substance that can strengthen any sickness: *stress*. What was the major stressor that helped jump-start your thyroid disease? I am quite sure this six-letter word kicked my butt to thyroid Hades.

Unquestionably, the medical community has given stress more respect in recent years, reporting that stress can intensify illnesses and, in some cases, kill. Just ask a cardiologist what stress can do. If this fact is recognized by so many, why do we ignore and/ or accept continuous stressful situations in our lives? Being the inquisitive person that I am, I began to analyze this phenomenon. I interviewed others to get their opinions about stress, watched documentaries, read articles, and so on. Then I checked to see what Mr. Webster had to say. *Ugh!* The dictionary's numerous definitions *stressed me out*. There are *fourteen* different definitions for the word *stress*. Weeding through all of those definitions—and then trying to decipher which one best fits the classification of something that could result in death or disease—caused me to do what I do best after a stressful situation: *take a nap.*

If my thyroid hormone levels are up or down either way, and I am faced with too many choices, I find myself heading down Berserk Boulevard. This is why we should continuously have our thyroid levels checked every three months (or sooner, if your doctor recommends it). So many of the non-thyroid afflicted, do not understand how difficult it is for us to make the right decision or any decisions at all, for that matter. To illustrate, it is like your brain is inside that head of yours, anxiously working away, literally trying to seek out a needle in a haystack. Once it finds the needle, the brain starts celebrating—"Yippee! Here it is!"—but the process was long and arduous. At my sickest, this simple question was like trying to locate that needle: "Ma'am, do you want paper or plastic?"

Before my thyroid diagnosis, I could never understand why that question from the store clerk would send me close to the edge. I knew making that decision was not rocket science, but it gave me trouble nonetheless. Every time! Somehow it didn't dawn on me that this question would be asked *during every purchasing event.* And understanding how simple a question it was, but also knowing that it caused so much deliberation, would perpetuate a dizzying effect. *If only they would give me the chance to sit down for a minute in the checkout aisle and contemplate which one I really needed . . . paper or plastic,* I would say to myself. Ha! Perhaps they should have a separate checkout lane for us, "Lane 2: The Thyroid Lane."

When the thyroid goes all wonky, so can the brain—and vice versa, I guess—because the thyroid and the brain are tight coworkers. After diagnosis and treatment, I continued to have problems with working through multiple choices. This was mainly because a thyroid that is not fully functioning does not give a person the essential nutrients needed for ample brain and body performance. Also, it is difficult for doctors to dial in the correct thyroid medication dosage to mimic a healthy functioning thyroid. So while doctors try to figure out how to reign in my rogue thyroid and immune disorder, I use my MacGraver tricks (for example, naps) to keep all my symptoms at a dull roar.

Two hours after my dictionary-induced nap, I woke up refreshed and ready for more stress education. I isolated the definitions with which most of us are familiar and that negatively affect us. *Whew!*

Here's my abridged version: *whatever causes pain, fear, emotional strain, or tension, both physical and mental, is stress.*

As much harm as stress can do to the human body, I really wanted good ol' Mr. Webster's *first* description, out of *all fourteen*, to say the following: "Stress is evil; do something about it. Grab it by the you-know-what, or you will be sorry. Sickness and disease will take over your life." This would have warranted a "Yea!" and a fist pump—and no nap.

The American Psychological Association reported in 2009 that 66 percent of surveyed adults had been told by their doctors that they have one or more chronic stress-related conditions (helpingpsychology.com, 2010). I believe most of us autoimmune disease sufferers would agree that stress was the main trigger that initiated our diseases. Stress is the kerosene thrown on smoldering coals that creates an inferno. Medical experts have often said that the daily personal anxieties we endure affect our dynamic trio: mind, body, and soul. Hey, think about this: *your* trio is not the only thing affected by stress; others in your path are affected as well because stress can be the gift that keeps on giving. Most of us aren't that skillful at maintaining calmness during highly stressful situations. We freely involve everyone—and who knows, maybe this contributes to the large number of chronic illnesses in our society. Wow, we all make each other sick. Isn't that great? Am I wrong? Look at my example below:

Hypothetical Example:

Pretend that stress is measured in *pounds*.

Your stressed-out friend calls you around 10:00 p.m., crying about a traumatic event going on in her life (three pounds). You listen intently, trying to be the good friend that you are, but your face tells a different story. You are rolling your eyes because this is the twentieth time she has been in this situation throughout your friendship. (It isn't necessary for me to detail the friend's circumstances in this hypothetical; you can insert your own drama-filled friend and his or her "situation," to paint yourself a better picture if you want.) You are quite curious as to how she has this enormous amount of desperation in her voice, as if this is the very first time she has ever been in this predicament. The first dozen or so times that you heard her rant, you made attempts to give advice, but now you have learned to respond by saying, "Uh, huh . . . Really, that's horrible." You manage to get off the phone by 10:30 p.m., which is a record. You are tired yet all wound up from the conversation. You and your husband are settling into bed together, and you start venting your frustrations to him about how exasperating your friend can be. You turn to your husband and ask, "What do you think I should do?" He says, "Huh?" He was not listening to a word you said (five pounds). The next morning you are tired and mad. Mad at your friend for being an idiot, mad at your husband for not listening, and mad at yourself for losing sleep over any of it. Pissed that your husband got to the shower before you, you head to your child's room to make sure he is getting ready for school, and he is. *Ahhhh, my baby,* you think. *This is the one bright spot in my life right now.* Until your child hands you a two-page permission slip, asking for pertinent medical information and money so he can attend a field trip. The bus will arrive in ten minutes, and the slip shows in big, bold letters that the deadline to turn it in is *today* (ten pounds). You head off to work—lots of weight to be added here:

- Rush-hour traffic: five pounds (Add another five if you are late or if there is inclement weather.)
- Just the act of pulling into the parking lot: two pounds
- The wait for the elevator: two pounds
- The walk toward your cubicle: ten pounds (Five pounds if you have an office, and if your office or cubicle is near the break room, add another ten pounds.)

I could write an entire book about *just* the cubicle—for making many people's lives a living hell. The creators of this horrid contraption should be doing ten to twenty in a cubicle of the concrete variety. Dilbert, the satirical office comic-strip cynic, and I are kindred spirits; the man just gets it. We both feel the same way about those darn gray boxes. Cubicles give off a false sense of security—like driving down the highway in a golf cart.

Forty or fifty years ago when cubicles came onto the office scene, the cubicle salesmen probably enticed management with the notion that they could shove numerous, smelly, obnoxious, gum-chewing, long-nailed, computer-clanking bodies into one room ergonomically and effectively. Guaranteed to get the *most* out of every employee . . . Yea!

If you are a cubicle dweller, this is your stress weight class:

- Tap on the shoulder to get your attention: ten pounds (twenty pounds if your neck hurts)
- Over-the-cube talker: five pounds
- The person who stands at your cube, silently waiting for you to notice: twenty pounds
- "I am going to set these papers down [at *your* cubicle] while I go to the bathroom": ten pounds (If they say "pee": fifteen pounds.)
- Your cubicle is Grand Central Station: thirty pounds (If you have to meet deadlines: fifty pounds.)

Add more work weight for IT issues, meetings, mandatory tornado drills, complainers, and visitor anxiety from management (thirty to fifty pounds).

After work, you make a stop at the grocery since you forgot to take the chicken out of the freezer to thaw for dinner because you were too busy in the morning making up fake dentist and doctor's telephone numbers for your child's permission slip. You have no idea where the school is taking your child; it could be to a strip club, for all you know.

While grocery shopping, you are able to find something healthier than pizza or fast food but not healthy enough to win you the Mother of the Year award. What your family eats is a big concern: five pounds.

The checkout lanes at the grocery go on forever: eight pounds.

Your stress weight is intensified by the checkout lady who feels the need to scan the items at a rate of one item per hour and then deems it important to strategically place the groceries in the bag as if she were placing a fragile, premature newborn in a car seat. "They are hash browns for crying out loud—throw those suckers in! *Geesh*." (Add ten pounds.)

Later in the evening, everyone in your household bears the brunt of the pounds of stress hanging from your shoulders. They pay the price, and you feel guilty. Guilt weighs a ton.

Take the above scenario and add other life stressors—environmental, food-related, spiritual, and so on. Why then are we shocked and amazed at signs of severe depression and anxiety (mental); headaches and stomach and digestive issues (physical); and discontentment (spiritual). And don't even get me started on the stress of getting repeatedly misdiagnosed. Years of living this way can most certainly lead to autoimmune diseases, especially if there is an underlying/subclinical condition lying in wait, *anticipating* stress weight.

Fifty million autoimmune disease sufferers in the United States and nearly two hundred million worldwide were perhaps oblivious to the fact that an enemy was awakened at the most inconvenient moment, rearing its ugly head, ready to strike. Strike with Hashimoto's, Graves', Crohn's, or type 1 diabetes. Then *BAM!* You are on medications for the rest of your life. Even after your diagnosis, allowing the weight of stressors to continue to pound on you can produce more illnesses or even kill you. Sadly, if enough weight is placed on even the sturdiest of structures, it will eventually break. I have no doubt my thyroid disease was borne from stress similar to that in the theoretical tale above, perhaps with a few extra pounds included.

Many of life's little stressors cannot be changed or avoided. What you *can* change is what I call the four Ps: your position, perspective, pressure, and pain.

Position: In season one of the television show, MacGyver narrowly escapes a car about to be smashed by one of those junkyard smooshers. Since he cannot flee from the side doors, he pries the backseat down and jumps out of the trunk in the nick of time.

MacGraver's Tip

Avoid drama-filled situations and nagging coworkers. Get up and take walks; move to an empty conference room to work, especially if it is imperative that you make looming deadlines. Take a break from high-maintenance friends. (Don't always take their phone calls.)

Perspective: MacGyver's peril on the television show is usually displayed with humor. While instructing a female heroine who is trying to stop deadly sulfuric acid from leaking by blocking the leak with chocolate candy bars, MacGyver tells her to make sure the chocolate melts on the acid and not on her hands.

MacGraver's Tip

Find the humor amid your stress. When you're dealing with the lady at the grocery, make up a funny story about why she is behaving that way. For example, she has a bomb strapped to her midsection. If she rings you up at a pace of two—items an hour instead of one, she and the entire store will blow to smithereens. Even Sandra Bullock could not save the day. With this viewpoint, you will be laughing in no time. Laughter takes some stress weight off.

Pressure: This is not always the best solution. It could backfire. However, on occasion, even MacGyver would have to use extreme force if necessary. It always amazed me how little scrawny Richard Dean Anderson could continually knock the bad guy out with just one punch.

MacGraver's Tip

Sadly, there are individuals who enjoy causing strife and stress for others. If you have tried most everything and there is absolutely no way you can completely avoid a person who is like this, then you must turn the tables on him or her. Fight fire with fire. For example, the next time your hubby tells you a long, drawn-out story, play the "huh" card. See if he likes it.

Pain: Although MacGyver's character was not super muscular, I am sure Richard Dean Anderson had to stay in shape to play that role. It takes a lot of energy to pull off some of those MacGyver-like tricks.

MacGraver's Tip

Get your pain from somewhere else. Exercise is a wonderful stress reliever, so forget about everything that you have ever felt about exercise and think of it as a new survival technique. A symptom of most autoimmune diseases can be extreme amounts of joint and muscle pain. After my radiation, the joint pain did not subside. I chose to go through physical therapy so that I could perhaps pick up some helpful tips to ease the pain. It worked. I do these short, but effective exercises every day:

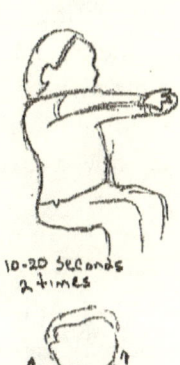

10-20 seconds
2 times

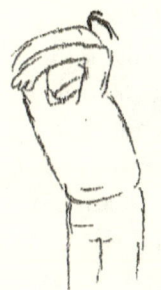

8-10 seconds
each side

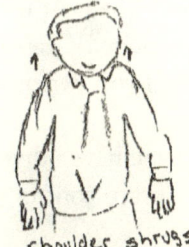

shoulder shrugs
3-5 seconds
2 times

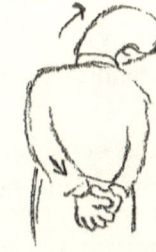

10-12 seconds
each arm

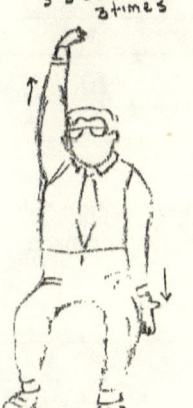

8-10 seconds
each side

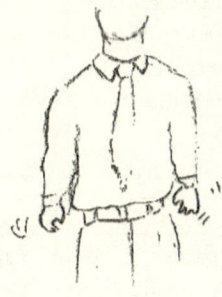

shake out hands
8-10 seconds

Once you are able to get your body conditioned to the point that it is stretched out enough for the pain to subside, you can then start an exercise regimen.

The thyroid regulates serotonin, norepinephrine, and gamma-aminobutyric acid, all of which contribute to normal brain functioning. So, when the thyroid is malfunctioning and your condition is not thoroughly controlled by medication, stress is magnified. When this occurs, there is no telling how a thyroid sufferer's will react to any stressor, let alone a major one.

I love grids and visual illustrations; you will see a lot of them in this book. Grids are great for those with thyroid problems because our cognitive abilities are somewhat diminished. At times, if information given to us is not compact and concise, it gets lost in the vast wasteland in our brains; and let me tell you, when it is lost . . . it is lost forever.

Please take note of the following stress grid. If you have a thyroid condition, these symptoms can be extreme and hard to control.

Stress Warning Signs and Symptoms	
Cognitive Symptoms	Emotional Symptoms
• Memory problems • Inability to concentrate • Poor judgment • Seeing only the negative • Anxious or racing thoughts • Constant worrying	• Moodiness • Irritability or short temper • Agitation, inability to relax • Feeling overwhelmed • Sense of loneliness and isolation • Experiencing Depression or general unhappiness
Physical Symptoms	Behavioral Symptoms
• Aches and pains • Diarrhea or constipation • Nausea, dizziness • Chest pain, rapid heartbeat • Loss of sex drive • Frequent colds	• Eating more or less • Sleeping too much or too little • Isolating yourself from others • Procrastinating or neglecting responsibilities • Using alcohol, cigarettes, or drugs to relax • Developing nervous habits (e.g. nail biting, pacing)

Bottom line, a stressful situation can either come at you like a speeding bullet or like a piece of lint gently drifting in your direction, softly landing on your lapel. Either way it makes an impact. Learn how to recognize this unwelcomed visitor by taking inventory from the *stress signs and symptoms* grid. If you are feeling too much stress weight, remember the four Ps and put them into practice. Don't forget, my thyroid-ailing brothers and sisters, this is not about being mean, self-centered, or antisocial. This is about survival.

―

Coming Attractions

In the next chapter, I will tell the story of how the weight of stress triggered my own thyroid autoimmune disease (Graves' disease). My evolution into physical and mental decay was inconceivable. How could someone in her late thirties experience all these symptoms? My deep desire is to help other thyroid-disease sufferers (diagnosed or undiagnosed) understand that they are not alone. If my story sounds familiar to you, seek help immediately. If you are met with a lot of balking and resistance, keep searching until you find the health-care practitioner who will listen and treat you effectively. I can't *stress* this enough.

**And now a word from one of my MacGraver friends, Sherri, who has Crohn's disease.

I take inspiration from a book that says, "Under any circumstances always do your best, no more and no less. But keep in mind that your best is never going to be the same from one moment to the next" (*The Four Agreements: A Practical Guide to Personal Freedom* by Don Miguel Ruiz).

I am working on remembering my best is defined by whether I'm sleeping well or exhausted, my symptoms are flaring or I'm feeling well, and gauging my emotions—angry, content, jealous, happy. These affect how high the bar is set for me daily (sometimes hourly). When I remember that, I feel less guilt on what I'm not getting done—the should'ves, would'ves, could'ves. And isn't guilt what causes us the most physical harm in the end?

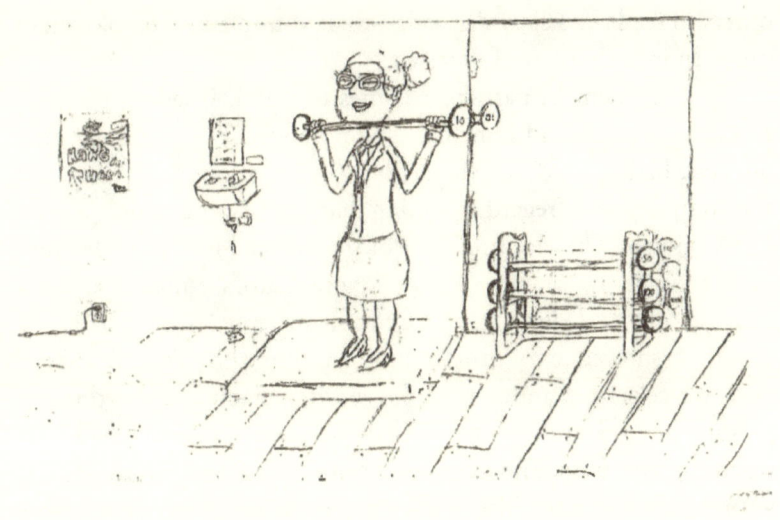

Chapter 2

My Stress, The Pit

I apologize in advance! Forgive me for droning on about my personal stress experience in this chapter. If you would be so kind, though, indulge me for one moment, as I feel it is important to explain how compounded stress claimed a piece of my essence—essence that shifted me from sanity to psychosis!

I used to consider myself a mentally tough person before thyroid disease. Never let them see you sweat? Ha. I didn't sweat . . . *ever.* But then my icy disposition cracked and shattered into a million pieces after I became an employee at . . . Umm . . . Okay . . . See here's the thing, I was going to *name* my old employer—the place that caused me so much turmoil and pain—until a friend of mine informed me of the potential for a libel lawsuit. Buzz kill. Serious days of contemplation followed after I got this advice. I really want others to see how a slow drip of stress at your place of employment can turn into a gusher of illnesses.

One incident in particular comes to mind. I had sent a mass e-mail to several head honchos. The note was about a change that our state had enacted, which greatly affected various departments in the company with regard to billing and claims processing . . . you know, money. The vice president of the hospital replied to *everyone* in the e-mail by saying, "Please ignore Carol's e-mail and don't respond." Now, I don't think he meant to reply to all, but in any event, it showed two things: his stupidity and his callousness. Several weeks later, another employee with an actual title—director of something or other—forwarded the *same* message I had sent regarding the state, and responses came firing back from various figureheads who acted like (a) they had never heard this news before and (b) a catastrophic fire needed to be extinguished. Some were even mentioning how getting this "late" news was going to put their respective departments behind the eight ball. I quickly found out that demeaning employees was a common, everyday practice for these folks. Even if it really was not my place to be the bearer of such news, the situation could have been handled differently. I never heard from anyone before or after that incident about whether distributing e-mail of that nature was restricted only to bigwigs. The ice water in my veins began to boil.

Why management chose and accepted this condescending culture, albeit unconsciously (I hope), to that enormous degree was beyond me. I realize there is a certain culture in *every* workplace; the leaders usually dictate the atmosphere. I've been a part of a variety of workplace cultures that ranged all the way from anarchy (the negative) to harmony (the positive). And I don't care how much money a person makes, working in a continuously negative atmosphere can be stressful. Some workplace environments offer the combination of negativity *and* tyranny; t*his*, my friends, can be detrimental.

A National Geographic documentary called *Stress: Portrait of a Killer* highlights many studies indicating how a person's hierarchy within a social environment can have a huge impact on their stress level. Doctors studied various species extensively and found surprisingly (at least for me) that the low man on the totem pole exhibited more stress than the dominant species. In the workforce, the dominant people are usually those with the superior titles. They *appear* to work more hours, are given more responsibilities, and often have more gray hair. The National Geographic study (done primarily on animals) showed a repetitive cycle of the dominant-ranking species picking on the lower species, which in turn pick on those that are even lower. The lowest of them all exhibited various illnesses, high blood pressure, increased heart rates, and in the case of rats, fewer brain cells.

Fewer brain cells! Hey, come on! You can't blame me for wanting to drag that unpleasant place of employment through the mud! Lawsuit? *Whatever*. Who cares?! The immense contempt I carried for that place was too strong; consequences be damned. But then I found out that my old company's name originated from a generous family who donated the land on which the facility stands. Disparaging the surname of those charitable donors who had bequeathed their property was not a part of my plan. They are off the hook, and I will *reluctantly* call them something else.

—

A new employee usually feels blissful and thankful on her first day—especially for a job that she sought rigorously. This is a typical feeling for most until mundane routines continuously encase the forty-hour workweek; and by then, the bloom is off the rose, as they say. Sadly, my rose never blossomed to begin with. I would have welcomed mundane; this place was anything but. Even unusual would have been tolerable. What greeted me at the . . . ummm . . . uh . . . The Bottomless Pit was nothing but chaos and dysfunction right out of the gate. On occasion, I would question whether this was a real functioning business or if, by chance, I had been unknowingly cast in a training documentary called *How Not to Run a Business*. Venting my frustrations to my friends and family would generate the same traditional response: "Every employer is like that!"

Have you heard this before? Don't you just want to slap the people who say this? It is moronic to give this supposedly reassuring response; how can anyone know what *every* place is like? Trying to set The Pit apart from all others, I always responded, "They are? Really? Every place has bloodsucking demons taking the souls of innocent people who just want a paycheck?"

Remember the movie *The Running Man* (1987) about a man, played by Arnold Schwarzenegger, who tries to survive attacks from inside a barbaric game show? Richard Dawson plays the sadistic host, throwing obstacles in Arnold's way, attempting to execute him before he can reach the finish. I believe Richard Dawson won an Academy award for this role. Anyway, *I* felt like Arnold's character—I was the running man—except that my company's game show-like pay structure looked more like this:

- $300 a week for humiliation and degradation
- $200 a week for allowing them to kick you around the office for a while
- Grand prize: 3 to 4 percent cost of living raise for the year and an extra half day of paid time off to do whatever you want (For this, they take your soul and stick it in the paper shredder!)

Oh, and since life is just one big ball of irony, you should not be surprised to hear this "employee-enriching" company was a mental health facility. Yep, that's right. Throughout my tenure at The Pit, I worked in administration, which meant no client contact; however, I would venture to guess that spending eight hours with the unpredictable, mentally ill clients would have been easier.

Sticking with pseudonyms, I'll call my old boss Jester (Jes for short). Jes was an amiable elderly man with an entertaining sense of humor. His personality was a cross between Michael Scott from *The Office*, Robin Williams, and Don Knotts. He resembled a skinny, gangly Ernest Borgnine. He was not at all attractive, yet he always had a bevy of the prettiest office chicks surrounding him. They loved his humor, and he loved to perform. I often heard from his harem how lucky I was to have Jes as a boss. "Yeah, lucky," I would say, trying very hard to sound sincere. People need to realize that *working* for Bozo the Clown is quite different from hanging out with him at the water cooler. It was difficult to get anything done; he was full of nonstop folly. I wanted to laugh with him—and ram paper clips up his nose all at the same time. Cognitive dissonance can certainly magnify stress.

On my first day of the job Jes warned me about his memory problems. *Of course you can't remember things*, I thought. He looked every bit of eighty years old. Many months later, I found out he was only sixty. There were a lot of contradictions with this man. His hobbies included playing with pivot tables in Microsoft Excel, yet he was not nerdy. He was a churchgoer with the worst foul mouth I had ever heard. It meant nothing to him to drop a few f-bombs, anywhere, anytime, around anyone. He complained the company was always in the red, yet he was constantly upgrading his pay grade. Oh, wait . . . He was the CFO, so that is not really a contradiction in today's corporate world—more of a foregone conclusion.

Jester approached me one morning to ask if I would make copies for an upcoming presentation to the board of directors of the hospital.

"Carol, can you make ten copies for me, my dear?"

"Sure, do you want them stapled?"

"Yes, thanks. That would be fine."

A few minutes later, I gave him the copies collated and stapled. He asked me to lay them down on the corner of his desk. I set them down and walked back to my cubicle.

Two hours later . . .

"Carol, can you make ten copies for me? I need to do a presentation for the board of directors."

I started laughing because this old dude is rarely, if ever, serious; but when he looked at me like there was something wrong *with me*, I realized this senile man was totally serious.

"Ummm, I already made them . . . I—I put the papers on your desk." Since this was a new employee-boss relationship, I was trying to do my best to sound benevolent.

"You did?" Jes was genuinely confused.

Immediately, I jumped up and started walking to his office, still halfway expecting him to shout out, "April Fools!" or "Psych!" or *something*! We both entered his office and damn if I did not see those papers. I snatched the originals out of his hands, without a word, not caring if I assaulted him with numerous paper cuts, and stomped to the copier. Surely, the rest of the office and probably a few floors down could hear me angrily clacking on the copy machine. I came back with the papers and laid them down on the same freaking spot they had been on previously.

"Oh, hon, I need them stapled," said Jester.

In my anger, I had forgotten to staple them. Growling, I went back and stapled them manually instead of having the copy machine do it—like I'd done *the first time*!

"Here you go."

"Great! Thanks, you rock . . . We have the makings of a great relationship, baby."

To this day, I have no idea where those originals went.

This would have been an amusing "Groundhog Day" moment except for the fact that dealing with people who have memory issues has *always* been my biggest pet peeve. I know what you are thinking, thyroid sufferer: this episode was possibly a preview into *my* future. Dealing with this man's senility, I'm sure, was a lesson for me somewhere. But I wasn't getting it at the time; all I received from him back then was a headache. I had no idea that one day my once near-perfect memory would resemble that of my old boss Jes.

His memory problems and his almost nonexistent work ethic continued with severity. If I gave you more examples, you probably would not believe me. I still don't believe it myself! The problem with having an inept manager is that he or she will notoriously blame the underlings if a mistake is made. Jes did this often. The more I tried to defend myself, the more I looked like the bad guy because everyone just loved foul-mouthed, fun-loving Jester. The weight of stress and its effects started to show very soon after my employment.

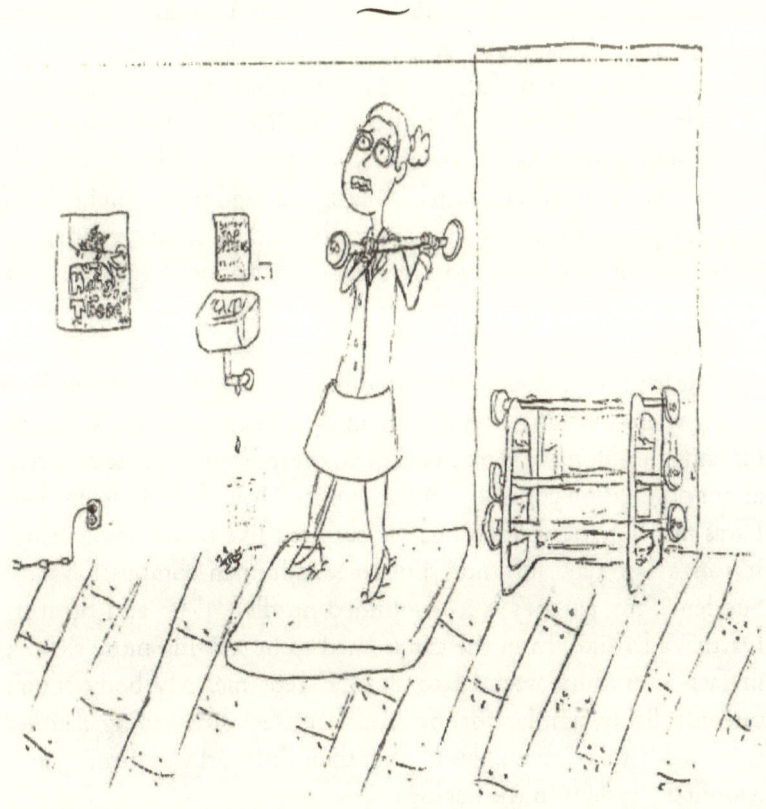

It was a yearly tradition for me and my husband to spend the weekend at a nearby gambling casino with family to celebrate his birthday. The casino was only a two-hour drive—not far, but we made it a long getaway weekend. A comfortable yet characteristically gaudy hotel was connected to this casino. We would commandeer five or six rooms on one floor for the entire weekend, and two of them had to be adjoining; those two rooms were dubbed Party Central. This yearly retreat yielded nothing but fun and relaxation, despite whether or not the house won!

On Saturday mornings, you might find each member of the Party Central Gang doing what he or she wanted. My husband could be found lying poolside all day; my sister and her spouse liked to visit local wineries. I was flexible. On one particular excursion, I decided to ride along with my mom and dad to a nearby horse racetrack. It was a scorching-hot day. As I climbed into the backseat of their old-fashioned, stylish black Cadillac, the darkness of the car created a sauna-like atmosphere. My dad promptly cranked the air on high, sympathetic to what black, baking leather might do to his baby girl's legs. The air instantly felt good. A Saturday morning drive with mom and pop, lots of great conversation . . . it felt like it was going to be another drama-free Party Central weekend. Or so I thought.

I dearly love my papa, but he would drive *about ten miles an hour* to anywhere—on any stretch of road. I had become accustomed to his chugging along, but on this day, an overpowering desire to arrive at our destination controlled my thoughts. Heavy breathing ensued; I was nearly hyperventilating. My skin felt like it was smoldering. It *was* a hot day, just not spontaneous-human-combustion hot! Suddenly, my parent's voices sounded muffled, deep and breathy, Darth Vader-like. Even the car seemed to be moving more slowly; in fact, everything seemed to slow. Except me. My body shook uncontrollably, similar to how your legs feel after riding a roller coaster. My folks were unaware that their little girl was turning into Mount St. Helens in the backseat.

Cheerful dialogue with my folks moments earlier suddenly shifted into me giving them a faint "yeah" or "uh-huh" every now and again. Trying to keep Helen dormant was unsuccessful; she, unfortunately, had other plans. Her eruption arrived with a bloodcurdling cry, "ROLL DOWN MY WINDOW NOW!" The temperature in the air had nothing to do with my behavior; it was my own body going haywire.

My dad rolling the backseat window down for me was the fastest I had ever seen him move, bless his heart! My conniption in the car concluded with me thrusting my head out the window, sweating and panting like a bloodhound tracking an important scent. The locals got a nice show that day, I'm sure. "Hey, look at the crazy lady pretending to be a dog in that luxury car!"

I was hoping my backseat outburst was an isolated incident. So many questions spun around in my mind. *Was this a new female disorder? . . . Nah, no way—couldn't be.* I was way too young for any premenopausal permutation. Hot weather wasn't the culprit either. I was mostly in cool air; it had to be something else. Eventually I found out that it was an anxiety attack, and this was the just first of many attacks to come. I remembered hearing others discuss their own personal experiences regarding these types of attacks in the past; I used to question the authenticity of these accounts. "How in the world could a person's anxiousness cause some sort of body-gyrating attack? That sounds insane," I used to say.

~

MacGraver's Tip

Don't be judgmental! This practice always comes back to bite you in the butt!

~

Nonetheless, my parents and I brushed over the incident as if it had never occurred, which was fine with me; I was mortified. Sweeping the next panic attack under the rug was not that simple, as it took place when we arrived back at our hotel and stood inside the stifling five-foot-by-six-foot hotel elevator. This elevator crept along even more slowly than my pops, all the way to the twentieth floor. My parents had a full view of my trembling body this time; the sweat was pouring like I had just run a marathon. I racked my brain for a ruse. "Wow, I should have eaten more at the racetrack! Must be my blood sugar," I said. I don't think they bought it, but hey, it was

Party Central. The lie had to be accepted because the party had to go on!

I often replay that backseat incident over and over again, wishing that somehow, someway, someone could magically undo it! In my mind, that single event kick started my thyroid disease. In reality, however, my symptoms were present long before on a subclinical level. Still, I just can't help but feel that my illness chose that moment for its grand entrance. It said, "I hear there's a party . . . Where's it at?" Once an incurable disease crashes a party, it's one party crasher you can't get rid of!

Other attacks came soon after, primarily at The Pit. Being surrounded by those three gray partitions did not bolster my psyche, and attacks came on with great frequency. I was on the edge, losing it. Whenever Jester's wiry body would slink up behind me at my cubicle, he'd find me jumping sky high out of my skin. "What the heck do you want? What did you forget this time?" I could feel those words trying to force their way out, but I would refrain. Instead, our relationship evolved into me doling out nasty looks. But then he would say something funny, and I would laugh hysterically. He would walk away . . . and then I would start crying! I was not a crier. Heck, I wasn't much of a laugher either. I wasn't boring; I was just your typical, mellow, "I'd better check her pulse to see if she is still alive" kind of gal. Bipolar-acting Carol was all new to me. Coping with excessive behavioral changes while working and maintaining a household was at times unbearable. I never imagined a malfunctioning thyroid could wreak this much havoc.

―

Despite all the madness, I stayed at The Pit. The part-time hours were ideal; they allowed me to be there for my son when he got on and off the school bus. That was the *only* reason I tolerated Jes and the other misfit toys. I may sound like a bad mother, but sometimes I wonder if it was all worth it. Looking back, I realize now that I faced bullying on a corporate level. No matter a person's age, bullying is a nasty, ugly practice. My e-mails were continuously being ignored by mandate. Jes threw me under the bus whenever he could so that he wouldn't look bad. It was obvious, at least to me, that his insecurity about his age brought about his behavior. He wanted to get everyone to love *him*—not his work. If you loved good ol' Jester, then how could you fire him? I paid the price for his insecurities. I was the *only* one he managed in our two-person department. He left me to flounder, while he performed stand-up in the break room. If there was a major crisis, Jes had a great knack for sticking his head down in the sand; and the harder you pushed him to do something, the longer his head would stay down in that sand. No one had my back. I was alone—the kid on the playground no one picked to play with.

The next stressor came when a new psychiatrist was "hired" to work in our inpatient facility, covering for the other tenured doctors on weekends and holidays. I am going to call this person, Dr. Duh. One particular Pit doctor met Dr. Duh at a mutual friend's cocktail party. The two struck up a conversation and realized they were in the same profession, except that Dr. Duh was unemployed at the time. The Pit doctor said, "Well, what do ya know? We need help at our hospital. Come work for us, covering various shifts." And that is how it happened, ladies and gentlemen. Do you understand my reason for saying he was "hired"? I wish I had the imagination to fabricate this story, but that is *truly* how Dr. Duh became an *employee* at our hospital.

So Dr. Duh showed up one day and started working, seeing patients, prescribing medication, and supervising subordinates. After all, he was a doctor, right? Dr. Duh had worked for about three months when suddenly it dawned on him that he wasn't getting a paycheck for his service. He contacted the hospital's human resources department; they said they could not help him and sent him to the behavioral health administrative secretary, who sent him to the CFO, Jes. The chief financial officer's head was stuck in the sand (as previously discussed), so he asked me to handle it. Of course all of this makes total sense, doesn't it? A peon was handling the following:

1. A psychiatrist walks in off the street and starts caring for patients. He is not an employee, nor has he signed a contractual agreement to practice at our hospital.

2. No one knows anything about this man, except for the person who offered him a job . . . ummm . . . during cocktails. And the drinking doctor has no authority to hire anyone.

3. None of Dr. Duh's credentials were checked. What male hasn't lied about his profession at a party?

4. This was a serious situation! Can you say . . . lawsuits, national media attention, or someone getting seriously hurt under his care? And who was asked to handle this? Me. Little ol' entry-level me! I WASN'T EVEN ALLOWED TO SEND IMPORTANT E-MAILS!

Since I was Dr. Duh's point person, he called me repeatedly. The word *stress* does not begin to cover what it was like dealing with that man. The monotone of his voice alone sent chills down my spine. Think Dr. Hannibal Lecter, only creepier.

For months he treated seriously ill patients, covering shifts the other doctors didn't want. The Pit did not have a problem with him working; they just had trouble paying. He would call me over and over with the same monotone murmur to ask why this had become a complicated situation. Most of my workday was spent putting him off in the hope that the powers that be would come to their senses. Given that I was the only one who had a brain at The Pit, I could foresee what might happen if they never paid the man.

His calls continued, sometimes more than once a day. I would listen to his long-winded drivel, only because I felt sorry for him and truth be told, I was a little frightened too. It developed into a game: he would check the status, and I would e-mail the bigwigs. It became imperative for me to use e-mail (even though I wasn't allowed . . . I think) to cover my butt. Repeated disregard from management produced frequent daydreams of me sitting on the witness stand in a courtroom pointing at Jes and shouting, "That's the man who did it! He wouldn't pay Dr. Duh!" Then Jes would do a stand-up routine. He would have the jury, the judge, and Dr. Duh laughing, and somehow the whole incident would be declared my fault. My daydream bubble popped.

A few more weeks passed with no responses from management. He threatened a lawsuit: still, nothing! It was like I was sending a chain letter to these idiots. Finally—and it was about time—Dr. Duh told me he was *not* going to work the upcoming major holidays for which he was scheduled: Thanksgiving and Christmas. With great pleasure, I sent this *new* message to the head honchos. The (super intelligent) vice president in charge of The Pit immediately responded to my boss, the CFO, with a simple message that read, "Take care of this!" How about that? My e-mails don't go directly to management's trash bin. This would have been my play from the beginning. What took you so long, Dr. Duh?

The daily idiocy I endured from the moment I leapt into The Pit was incredible. By then I had endured two years with Jester and The Pit crew. Along with the Dr. Duh issue, my thyroid problem was starting to rev up with intensity; its engine was ready for liftoff!

—

Stay tuned for the continuation of chapter 2, "My Stress." Will the weight of stress at The Pit exacerbate Carol's autoimmune thyroid disease? Will she climb out of The Pit or get rescued by a tall, dark, handsome stranger? Don't turn the channel—don't miss the exciting conclusion!

**Time for a quick commercial break from one of my MacGraver friends, Edwina, who lives with CREST syndrome.

Crest Syndrome is one of those rare ADs, so there aren't a lot of people I've found who I can talk to about the disease. What has helped me is that I do a lot of research on my disease, the dos and don'ts.

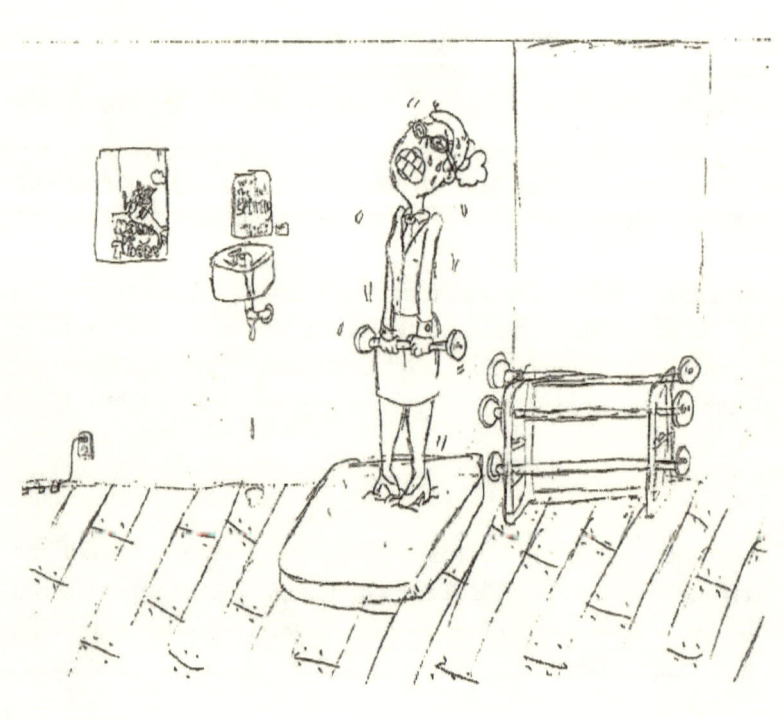

The Continuation of Chapter 2, "My Stress"

My symptoms were sporadic and not constant enough for me to Google a diagnosis. Physically, I would complain of fatigue, joint pain, and mild tachycardia. Those were issues I could overcome with a little rest and Advil; but my mental state during this time had become disconcerting. Going from having an even-keeled persona to being someone who, quite frankly, was unidentifiable scared the crap out of me. The experience was similar to the movie *Freaky Friday* except that those two gals switched into people with whom they were familiar. If all of a sudden I became my mother, I would know to laugh a lot, watch soap operas all day, cook, and be disagreeable. But I didn't know the person I was becoming.

The anxiety attacks were evolving from only occurring in close quarters to being full-blown social anxiety. Simple conversations with neighbors, family members, and friends about the weather could bring on severe attacks. Take, for example, this true incident involving my neighbor, who had only lived next door to me for about a month:

"Hi, Carol. How are you doing today?"

"Fine, how about yourself?"

"I'm doing great. It is a nice day today. What do you think the weather will be like tomorrow?"

This was about the time my brain acknowledged that a conversation was taking place, which caused my body to start trembling. Adequate responses usually came out of my mouth automatically at times like these; however, if I started to actually think about the current *conversation*, anxiety would set in. A flushing, hot sensation moved through me like a tidal wave. My voice did this Peter Brady crackle—and then the crying started. Yes, crying . . . about the weather. As this meltdown transpired, my neighbor looked at me, quite perplexed and awaiting my reply. My eyes were getting red and full.

"Ummmm, I am not sure . . . I better run—I have something cooking on the stove," I stammered. Then I darted in the house, narrowly dodging a smack into our storm door.

I was never a good liar, but how in the world could I have explained that having a conversation would result in a complete nervous breakdown right there on the front porch. I knew this preposterous problem had to be resolved. *I mean, really . . . I can't talk about the weather?* How was I supposed to work, go to family functions, or do *anything* where other people were involved? I knew could not live that way anymore.

My solution: I drank.

I do not believe I was an alcoholic, although some may disagree. The taste of alcohol never appealed to me. I did not love the buzz or high; it was just cheap medication to keep me functioning. That was all. It stopped my body shakes, trembling, and anxiety. Plus, as a bonus, I could cook or clean the house, as it also relieved my all-over joint pain. If there was no need for household chores or interacting with people, I didn't drink. In my mind, it was like chewing chalky Tums tablets: I hated the taste—it almost made me want to vomit—but it was medicine needed for indigestion. I refused to drink at work. The thought of getting caught smelling like a brewery terrified me. So I kept to myself. To avoid conversations there, I tried the "I'm on the phone" or "Oops, I have to run to the bathroom" tricks.

In hindsight I am not sure if it was the drinking or the progression of my disease (probably a little bit of both), but a new symptom began to emerge: paranoia. Jesse Ventura had nothing on me. I was convinced coworkers, friends, family members, and neighbors were all talking about me—like I was tabloid worthy or something. I was off my rocker. One particular day, probably after doing a couple of shots of "medicine," I decided to purchase a product called the Miracle Ear that I saw on a TV commercial. Only $19.95 plus shipping and handling: such a small price to pay to obtain all the proof I needed. Why I needed this proof and what I was going to do with it is beyond me.

My son and I were coming home from the store one day when I looked across the street and saw my two neighbors talking to one another. *Here is my chance to do surveillance*, I thought. I placed my boy in front of the television with a substantial snack. The work of a spy is time consuming. I was giddy with excitement and so proud of myself for remembering which junk drawer held the Miracle Ear. I would *finally* get to hear what my neighbors were saying about me! My investigative strategies involved a pretense of getting more groceries out of the car, and then secretly slipping down onto the floorboard. My five-foot-eleven frame scrunched down on the passenger side floor of my tiny Ford Focus. This wasn't pretty.

I don't know if my Miracle Ear was defective, but all I could hear was Sponge Bob and Patrick laughing and playing in Bikini Bottom. My son's cartoon was overriding all other noises—*CRAP!* Disentangling myself from the Focus, scratching and cutting up my legs in the process, I scampered back into the house to turn the sound down. It was not easy coming up with a good excuse to mute Sponge Bob. My son bought my explanation, so I ran back into the garage to resume my stakeout. Turns out, my Miracle Ear *was* defective. Or maybe this is the case with *all* "as seen on TV" products? I don't remember my Slap Chop behaving this way . . . Anyhow, all I heard was garbled, blowing wind. Unfortunately, I never got my proof. Looking back on my behavior, I wonder if seeing a therapist would have been beneficial. I don't believe I would have known what to say, though. I'd had a wonderful childhood and was living a great life as an adult; so I wasn't trying to drink for escapism. How could I tell someone that several months ago, I *had been* fine, but now, without any head trauma or major disease diagnosis, I had become unstable and had to drink to function? Was there a precedent for this? I was too paralyzed with fear to tell anyone what was happening to me.

—

Three years later, I was still working with potty-mouthed, politically incorrect, joking Jester. He had worn my nerves so razor thin that it was imperative to keep my distance. This was a defense mechanism. Avoiding Jes wasn't all that hard, though; it was easily accomplished by staying clear of his office or his main stage, the break room. Regrettably, my own stupidity put me up close and personal with Jes one day. It all began when Jes sent an e-mail informing me about a cubicle move that was to take place in a week. My new Pit place was going to be next door to the man whom some in the office called my boyfriend. To me, he was my stalker. I absolutely could not take any additional stressors, and I knew sitting next to this man might be the catalyst that would send me to one of our patient beds. I never figured out why he was infatuated with me. He was a middle-aged man, five feet tall, with long, mullet-style rocker hair—oh, and no teeth. He would constantly quote wrestling terminology. Who knew they had their own language? He liked to mimic Hulk Hogan's voice while yelling directly in my ear "Bring on the pain!" or "You can't see me!" How in the world could I get a double dose of crazy with Jes and Stinky Weasel Teeth and make it out alive? Stinky Weasel Teeth or SWT is not a pseudonym I made up for this book; it was the name I affectionately called him (behind his back). Mean, I know; but my son was into Ren and Stimpy at the time and the name fit.

Stinky Weasel Teeth and I became acquainted when he caught me one morning after Jes's 9:00 am comedy set in the break room. I was a new employee at the time, so I hung in there to make a good impression by laughing loudly at his performance. When his routine was finished, Jes left the room, slinking out with a couple of giggling office hotties. A few other Pit employees lingered, myself included. The water cooler had all my attention; I had to get the workday's H_2O intake, and my back was turned to those in the room who were still carrying on conversations. Suddenly I heard scattering footsteps fly out of the north and south exits. Everyone vanished. I turned around to see if I had missed an important drill of some kind. Instead, it was my first glimpse and whiff of SWT. My initial thought: *This is an office professional?* But despite his looks and scent (stale cigarette smoke and alcohol), he seemed very intelligent. I found out he was an army veteran who was fluent in several languages. I must have caught him on a bad day; he was crying (yes, crying) about how bad his back was hurting and how the pharmacy refused to fill his prescription for painkillers, which he had tried to refill again prior to the accepted refill date. I stuck around and gave him a sympathetic ear for what seemed like hours, no doubt propelling our relationship into what *he* later viewed as us being "soul mates." My only saving grace from having to hear daily stories about his back pain or his passion for wrestling was that we were on opposite sides of the building. It was apparent that being a Pit survivor would mean avoiding the break room altogether; no comedy or crying was fine with me. But now, a full eight-hour day of SWT? *Ugh.* Envisioning SWT shouting wrestling jargon in my ear while I attempted to work led me to promptly e-mail my boss Jes the following note:

> *Hey Jes, there is no way I can sit next to my "stalker" he would continuously bug me all day. I would need fly swatters and repellents just to be able to get any of my work done. If I have to endure this, I will slit my wrists making a bloody mess on the floor. I am sure you don't want that to happen. Hahaha.*

This was my feeble attempt to match my boss's buffoonery . . . you know, *speak his language.*

The next morning, Jes came wriggling over to my cubicle. I would bet money this dude did not have vertebrae, which would explain why he never defended me to the other managers—you'd have to have a backbone for that. Jess had a printout of my e-mail in his hand, and he asked me to come with him to human resources. *Are you kidding me?* I thought. He wasn't. Jes was wearing a rare humorless expression. In fact, he was almost unrecognizable.

With hesitation, I slowly got up from my seat and followed him to HR, which was on a different floor. We took the stairs instead of the elevator. For a split second, I was glad he had chosen the stairs. Seeing the big red EXIT sign in the stairwell was like a direct order coming from my consciousness. *Exit, Carol. Get the heck out of there!* I thought. *This is so stupid. Jes can say, do, and act anyway he wants, but now I have to go directly to the firing squad without a chance to explain myself.* I was getting angry.

We walked into the office, and the HR director of behavioral health was waiting for us. She quickly ushered us back into her office. I could not believe there were no big burly men with lab coats at the ready. I mean, really, their extreme attitude toward the situation was outrageous, especially, considering that they let Dr. Duh, (a man off the streets) *treat patients*. Here I am, bantering with Jester, and I get ostracized. I think the HR chick must have known of Jes's reputation, because surprisingly, after I explained my e-mail to her, she directed most of her attention toward Jes. She expressed the need for him to establish appropriate communication protocols with his employees. Jes looked at her blankly, as if he had no idea what she was talking about. Seeing him get lectured like that was my one and only bright moment at The Pit, which should give you an indication of the suck level.

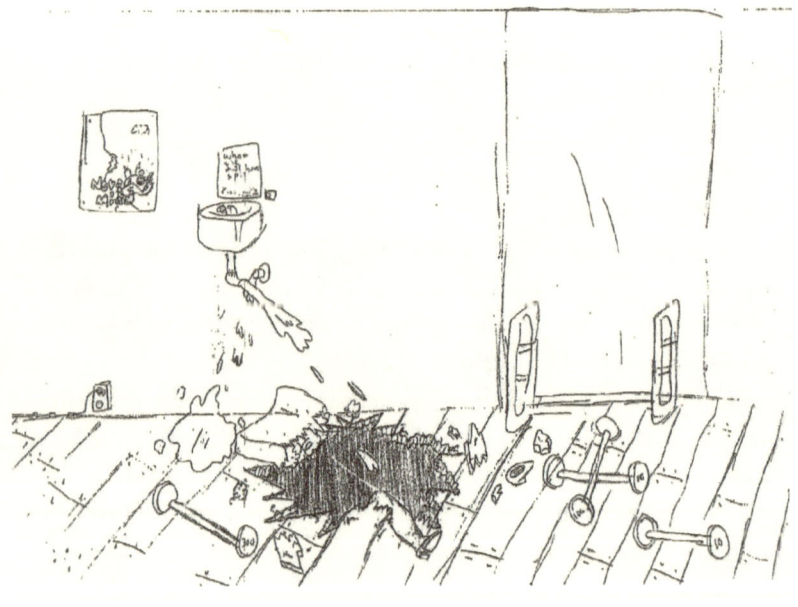

By this point, extreme fatigue had become a daily feeling for me. Performing minimal everyday tasks felt like trudging through mud. An energy level like that goes beyond being tired. In my younger days I worked the third shift, so I know what tired feels like. Tired means consuming a cup or two of caffeine and then being able to *fully* function for another eight to twelve hours if need be. But caffeine would not cut this coma-like condition. Everything was exhausted—my brain, my body, even my desire for accomplishments. When your desire is fatigued, being forced to function (go to school, work, etc.) makes you irritable. Going to bed around the same time as my grade-schooler was the norm. Ten to twelve hours of sleep each night didn't have any effect. Years in a coma would probably have worked, but I would not have wanted to test that theory.

—

Despite the lunacy (remember, I am talking about the employees) at this behavioral health facility, I worked my butt off. I come from military parents who taught their children to work hard in any situation. For years it was common for me to receive the typical 3 to 4 percent—*cough*—cost-of-living raise. Now it was time for my soon-to-be fourth and final Pit annual review. Well, unbeknownst to me, they changed the format of the performance review; this was not explained to me by my manager. Imagine that.

There I was bitching like I normally did about the conditions at The Pit because, of course, management had stressed that "a performance evaluation is the one chance to voice your opinions." Well, come to find out, if you bitched on the new performance appraisal, it was considered a reflection on you and only you. After my unknowing act of self sabotage, Jes gave me a 2 percent raise. This calculation, Jes explained, was based on the "scientific scoring" he was "instructed" to use for the latest performance appraisal format. Whatever. I am not sure if this was a *real* reason or a typical CFO explanation for the puny increase. But, unlike Dr. Duh, I was not going to continue working for what I considered "free." The next day, I submitted resumes to a number of different jobs—anywhere from positions pertaining to my degree all the way to folding towels in the hospital laundry room. I was getting out, and *finally* I did.

I scaled the wall out of The Pit, but the damage had been done. My symptoms were now in full force. There was no question that it was time for a diagnosis, and I at last got one.

I guess I also should mention that, during all this time, I was in my late thirties, was caring for a family, and had returned to school to obtain my college degree. My husband had become addicted to prescription painkillers. My son, who was considered "gifted," had decided it was much cooler to treat his school as a social-networking facility instead of a place to further his education; and my dad had been diagnosed with prostate cancer. I could have mentioned all of this earlier. I just really, really wanted to complain about The Pit and get that off my chest. *Man*, was that cathartic.

My point is that life happens. As you can see, life surely happened for me. It happened like a *two-hundred-ton freight train*. I am really not a moral-of-the-story kind of gal, but if I had known that allowing so much weight to pile up on me could possibly result in a chronic illness, I would have found help throughout this locomotive lunacy.

McGraver's Tips

Don't go it alone. Find support groups, books, and classes on dealing with difficult situations (such as drug-addicted husbands, difficult bosses, and uncooperative children). I am sure there was a perfect person out there who could have coached and/or mentored me in how to deal with some of these issues. Don't be afraid to seek help.

Let *out* what is in. Talk and breathe. *Talk*: I have found a lot of support from my peers on Facebook and Twitter. This is called "getting by with a little help from your friends" twenty-first-century style. And it works. *Breathe*: Mediation and breathing exercises work tremendously. A former coworker and good friend, who is also a mental health therapist, recommends daily meditation and breathing exercises. She explains, "It's a process of letting go mentally of some of our daily stressors."

Practice BLAH—no blame, no animosity, and no hard feelings. Negative actions only feed stress. My experience at The Pit was exasperating to say the least.

But harboring resentment is nothing more than playing the ugly horror movie over and over again in your head. Scientists who study the brain believe that humans do not have filters on the subconscious level to distinguish between what is real or imagined, so everything is perceived to be real (inwardquest.com, 2009). If a situation is terrible and beyond your control, move on to bigger and better things.

**And now for a short interruption from one of my MacGraver friends, Jaime, who has fibromyalgia and celiac disease.

"For me I am able to cope with my fibromyalgia with exercise. I know that sounds crazy since it is a pain disease, but for me it is the only thing that helps relieve the pain. I do mostly low-impact cardio and circuit training with light weights. I also feel really good after I have been swimming.

"Also, I see a massage therapist two times a month. Each time I go in I tell her where my pain is the greatest, and she works on that area. I usually leave feeling much better. I also take hot apple cider baths three to four times a week. I use about one quart of apple cider vinegar in my bath and soak for at least fifteen minutes but usually for thirty. It really helps loosen my muscles and relax them. Lastly, I started stretching/meditating to relaxing music each day after my workout. That helps me clear my head and focus on something other than the pain."

Chapter 3

Finally, Treatment!

Sitting in the hospital, waiting to be called back to take the radioactive pill, I began to think of the pretentiousness of hospital waiting areas nowadays. Hospitals contract with premiere design agencies to swank up their façades, but a stark contrast lies behind many of the various doors I see hospital staff hurry in and out of. Those rooms don't have color patterns and designs reminiscent of a Hilton hotel. Is it a ploy? A trick? An attempt to deceive me into thinking that what's behind door number one or two isn't really a house of horrors filled with barbarians and their instruments? (Did I mention my paranoia?)

"Carol." The nurse startled me out of my trance.

I got up slowly, as my body continued to ache from not being completely treated for my thyroid disease. The nurse smiled yet looked concerned, as though she were wondering why someone my age was moving at a snail's pace. She ushered me back to yet another waiting area. I had been through the hospital musical chair game before, though. They do love their little games.

"Someone will be right with you to take you back to another area," said the nurse.

"Thanks," I said politely even though I did not feel like bestowing such warmth. I felt like hell. And now my mood was shifting even more into a downward direction to match this new room's décor. There was nothing to look at in this waiting room, no peculiar statues of fish or cats staring at me. I was forced to think about me, my situation. I started going back.

How did I get here? Ten years of vacillating between feeling just okay and having various ailments: some, common; others, a great mystery. Visits to emergency rooms, urgent care facilities, and my primary doctor's office were becoming routine. It was tiring. But, fortunately, I had become an old pro at decoding doctors' faces. If they *thought* I had a sinus infection, I would receive the sympathetic look and antibiotics. Viral infections got a concerned look, along with the statement, "I think it is viral, but just to be on the safe side, I am going to write you a script for antibiotics." When I had one of my mysterious afflictions, this garnered a blank stare plus—you guessed it—a script for antibiotics.

Me: So, umm . . . You don't want to do any sort of blood or diagnostic testing? I believe this is my nineteenth infection in ten months.

MD: Uh huh . . . Well, if you get that twentieth infection, come back and see us. We may have to see what is going on with you, young lady.

I am waiting for the day a drugstore will offer this special: **AFTER YOUR FIFTH ANTIBIOTIC PRESCRIPTION FILL, GET A FREE YEAST INFECTION KIT!** The way drugstore pharmacies compete nowadays and since antibiotics are handed out like candy, this would be an ingenious marketing promotion, don't ya think?

The *unnecessary* thousands of dollars I spent on medical bills finally ended. My primary doctor had me undergo thorough diagnostic testing and lab work. The diagnosis came with a tremendous amount of relief: Graves' disease, a thyroid condition. My elation at this news may sound odd. A noncurable disease—*yippee!* But you have to understand that, after ten years of going around on this queasy curative carousel, I wanted off. This medical finding was justification, vindication, and satisfaction all in one.

If you are unable to relate, consider this scenario: you've taken your car to the mechanic a handful of times because you hear a knocking sound coming from under the hood. The mechanic cannot produce the noise when he drives your car around the block, so he keeps sending you on your way without a fix. Ten seconds after you drive away, the knocking starts again . . . *grrrrrr*. Several trips later, the mechanic finally hears the knocking and knows the problem. You experience a sense of relief—relief, even though the fix is a costly new engine.

MacGraver's Tip

When it comes to your health, be firm with your doctor. Explain that your continual bad feelings, both mentally and physically, are unacceptable. Firmness with facts is key. Keep a level head with doctors; high emotions have no place in their cold, emotionless patient rooms. Doctors like facts, figures, and timelines. (I have had a dry cough for x days). If they are unresponsive or unsympathetic, say, "*Sayonara!*" and search for another. I cried and threw temper tantrums on several occasions throughout those ten years, but that got me nowhere. Finally when I wrote down a list of my ailments, accompanied by timelines, my MD took notice.

My primary doctor recommended I see an endocrinologist, someone who specializes in thyroid diseases. Getting in to see almost any specialist, especially an endocrinologist, is incredibly difficult; however, after she viewed my grim test results she scheduled me right away. My results indicated one of the worst cases she had seen; charting an immediate treatment plan was imperative. She recommended a popular treatment for my condition called RAI, which stands for radioactive iodine. RAI treatment involves swallowing a radioactive pill typically given by a nuclear medical technician. (That doesn't even sound humane, does it?) I am now convinced that getting a pill from a nuclear medical technician is not a treatment for anything. It's more like torture. Nevertheless, I was mentally unstable, in extreme physical pain, and near heart failure. Heck, I would have taken a bubbling beaker from Vincent Price at that point. But still, as I sat in that hospital room, I kept asking myself, *How did I get here?* Hmmmm . . . perhaps it was:

> *pesticides, too many antibiotics(in food and in prescriptions), processed foods, bioterrorism, microwave ovens, high-fructose corn syrup, contaminated water, things made in China, trans fats, nuclear power plants, nutrient-deficient soil growing our fruits and vegetables, antibacterial soap, germ-infested shopping cart handles, global warming, diet drinks, smog, pollution, lipstick, water bottles, radiation from dental/medical X-rays, cell phones, insects, gluten, fast food restaurants, genetics . . . WHAT?!*

Once again, curious Carol went on a mission to understand why her body had to go all Rambo against itself. *This* search was less stressful. I didn't need a nap because no one has any idea how autoimmune diseases are acquired; there's not much information to weed through or analyze, if everyone is clueless. "No one knows" was written in just about every publication I came across, which pretty much leaves no room for further explanation or interpretation.

So, not only is getting a diagnosis like potty-training a two-year-old boy (nearly impossible), the medical community can't even tell us why our bodies decide to go rogue. I have heard many a sufferer say, "If you can't tell me how, then how much faith should I place on the medical community's treatment plan?" This is why many of us feel the need to scan the Internet for answers. Combing through blogs, social networks, and various medical sites satisfies an enormous hunger for knowledge. Docs hate this, though. Several of mine sternly advised me not to search the web for insight into my ailments. "It only makes you paranoid," they'd say. And if they see you with Internet literature in hand, you might as well prepare for a heavyweight boxing match. I've come to the realization that the only reason docs tell us not to do these types of searches is to keep us from finding out how much they *don't* know. I mean, come on, they went through a bazillion years of school, and all most of them can do well is write scripts for antibiotics.

"Carol."

Jarred once again out of another daydream, I added another fake smile onto my face. Here was my final escort, alas, the nuclear medical technologist. This one mumbled. I could not understanding most of what he said. Sigh, I should have known. This is what a Nuclear Medical Technologist was going to be like: no personality, monotone, soft spoken and slow talking—kind of like your typical IT guy. Looking down at the floor, he told me he had "another patient next door" and he would "be back shortly." He either said that or "A pastor is on the floor on his back. I am trying to get him up, but he is too portly." The first one sounds more feasible. I sat quietly and waited.

Another room with no abstract artwork to analyze. Boredom sent me into the black hole that is my purse to see how I could occupy my time. In my experience, slow-talking mumblers aren't swift in their movements. I knew I might be there awhile. I found a scrunched-up pamphlet that my endocrinologist had given me that briefly described the thyroid and explained its functions and what could go wrong with it. At that time, I did not want to read it—I was living it. The person who wrote the pamphlet had probably gone to school to gain their knowledge, but I felt that living it made me a better expert.

"*Ha!*" I laughed out loud, covering my mouth quickly, to shut myself up. I'm not sure why I was embarrassed, though; no one else was in the room. The first sentence in the pamphlet was quite humorous to me:

> *The thyroid gland is one of the most important of the endocrine glands.*

My body chose one of the most important glands to attack. *Way cool, body . . . You are such an overachiever.*

I continued reading:

The thyroid gland is shaped like a butterfly situated in front of the neck. The thyroid is responsible for controlling how the body uses energy, how protein is made, and most importantly how sensitive the body should be to other hormones, such as melatonin, serotonin, epinephrine, insulin, etc. The hormones that the thyroid directs are important to all other systems as well as other glands, namely the pituitary and the hypothalamus, which are situated in the brain. All these working together are needed for fluid bodily function. Because of the importance of this gland, over or under active functioning from this gland produces a myriad of symptoms. (Tell me about it.)

The mumbler returned. He came down to sit across from me in his long white lab coat. He was more official looking than everyone else at that hospital: no spots or blemishes on his lab coat, pristine khakis, and not one scuff mark anywhere on his shoes. Now, if he would just open his mouth to talk . . .

His mumbling really had my mind racing in all sorts of directions. The more he mumbled, the more my mind twirled with thoughts.

I stared at his lips because they were so chapped I wondered if they were hurting him. Then I began looking at his freckles and made designs on his face with an imaginary marker. I felt it was fine to stare at him like that because he kept looking down at the floor. I'm pretty sure he had no idea I was playing games with his face. He shocked me suddenly when he asked me a question—at least I think he did, because he paused and finally looked me right in the eye.

I cleared my throat. "I'm sorry, could you repeat that please?"

I believe he asked me if I had made arrangements to stay away from friends and family for at least three days.

"Yes," I answered. *Geesh, wasn't public speaking a part of his training?* This man was an American; he did not have a thick accent. Hmmm, I guess he just did not feel like opening his mouth to talk. *THEN, YOU KNOW WHAT, YOU SHOULD NOT HAVE THIS*

JOB! Just give me the pill, you thyroid assassin . . . I am getting agitated. He continued to mumble. I had to calm myself down.

Graves' disease is a form of hyperthyroidism. The name explains it all, "hyper" means everything speeds up: heart rate, emotions, thinking, etc. If I got too upset, my heart rate would speed up to the point that it literally felt like my heart was going to jump out of my chest. And the slightest little detail could get me going into a tizzy. *Ugh, I don't want to be escorted to yet another room with heart monitors and cathodes. Been there, done that.* I once needed *the jaws of life* to peel those cathodes off my skin—*ouch! Must calm down, Carol. Think about something else.*

I began to think about one of my interesting college courses where I learned about many Eastern religions. Several of them (for example, Hinduism, Sikhism, and Buddhism) accepted the doctrine of reincarnation. They believed that some humans are on an eternal incarnation cycle. They come back over and over again, either by choice—to learn and evolve—or as a punishment for a past life. If this were true, then I figured I used to be Attila the Hun. Or maybe I had ordered this disease along with all the accompaniments off the reincarnation menu in an effort to, in fact, learn and grow. I began picturing myself walking up to God and asking Him for the deluxe menu.

"My last life was boring and dull; I want a lot on my plate, God."

"Okay. Have you already been to Housewares and the Kids', Men's, and Education departments?"

"Yes, I just need to order my disease, and I'll be all set. A couple of angels told me I needed to see the Main Man for that."

"Now, are you sure you don't have to have a disease?"

"I spoke to Gabriel, and he said if I grab a doozy of a disease, I can really prosper in my *next* afterlife."

"He is right. Let me suggest an autoimmune disease."

"What is that?"

"It is not well known, but it will become an epidemic someday."

"Okay, let me take a look at the menu . . . Hmmm, this sounds interesting. I will take the Graves' disease. It seems the thyroid is a very important gland. I can't wait to see how jacked up I am going to be with this illness. Woo-hooo!"

"Okay, Carol, here is your menu. Good luck, my child."

Menu: Graves' Disease

Appetizer

- Heart palpitations
- Chronic sinusitis
- Allergies
- Allergy-related asthma
- Fatty lumps on various parts of the body
- Menstrual issues
- Digestive problems
- Mild joint pain

Main Course

- Heart palpitations leading to catheter ablation procedure that won't work, causing a max out on a prescribed beta blocker. Continue to have extreme tachycardia until thyroid treatment. Afterward tachycardia will be intermittent.
- Chronic sinusitis leading to sinus surgery to gut out the diseased sinuses. Continued sinusitis after surgery until proper thyroid treatment.
- Menstrual issues leading to a D & C, two ablations. None will work. Will have to wear adult underwear called Depends during periods.
- Body pain leading to twenty physical therapy sessions, many orthopedic appointments, and cortisone shots. Many chiropractic appointments until insurance stops paying.
- Serious digestive issues because the thyroid controls how food is metabolized.

Dessert

- Mental illnesses. Most MD's won't know a darn thing about this mainly because there will always be continuous arguments on mental illnesses and how they are treated.
  - Paranoia
  - Erratic mood swings
  - Suicidal thoughts
  - Psychosis

"Sounds great, God. If I am unable to learn and grow from all those ailments, which will systematically break down my body for many, many years, costing me a lot of money and my sanity, then I don't know what will!"

"That's the spirit, Carol! Now go and put your disease to good use."

As this dude kept rambling on about this poisonous pill and what I could expect as side effects, I nodded, but my daydreaming continued. I began to get angry with myself for ordering all those ailments from the Graves' menu. Maybe I should have passed on dessert? *AHHH, oh my goodness! What in the world am I thinking about? I am a Christian—I don't even ascribe to this philosophy.* I tell ya, the mind is a dangerous place when you are in the wonderful world of hyperthyroidism. I am getting angry about the fact that there is no ostentatious artwork in this stark room, about his mumbling, about a religion I don't even believe in . . . *DUDE, JUST GIVE ME THIS PILL ALREADY before I start believing little green men from another planet caused me to go haywire.* He must have heard my thoughts, or maybe he saw my feet getting antsy. I was tapping my foot at a rate of one hundred taps a minute, and since he was mainly looking down, he probably read toe-tapping instead of faces. He got up and walked over to the refrigerator to get the pill.

Ten years and it was all coming down to me just getting this one little pill. It was mind boggling. Could this have been anymore anticlimactic? I knew how Dorothy from *The Wizard of Oz* felt. All she had needed to do was click her freakin' heels. She could have avoided the evil monkeys, the scary dwarfs, and the talking forest creatures. I felt like Dorothy. Why couldn't my cardiologist, orthopedist, primary care doc, otolaryngologist, OB-GYN, or gastroenterologist have told me to click my heels? Instead, they all gave me Band-Aids for my issues and took a big chunk out of my wallet.

Before he opened the stainless steel refrigerator where the pill was housed, he put on a pair of large, white, elbow-hugging gloves. He pulled a matching silver canister, similar to a thermos, out of the silver refrigerator. The smokiness from the fridge was a little unsettling. Hmmm, maybe my space alien theory was right and only a pill from outer space could save me . . . The whole scene was beginning to look like something from *Star Trek*. He put the harmless-looking pill in a small white cup. There was no hint of it being radioactive; it just looked like a vitamin. I swallowed the pill, heard some more mumbling, and then he took off. That's it! My thyroid assassin did not leave me with any sage words like "May the force be with you" or "Change is the essential process of all existence." I'm not too sure, but I don't think I got any of that from him. *Oh well. The damage has been done. The poisonous pill is down. God give me strength.*

Because I was now radioactive, it was recommended that I stay away from my family for a few days. Soon after taking the pill, I decided to stay at a hotel situated just minutes from the hospital. I checked in during the early afternoon hours; my microwave personality was hoping that this pill would kill my overactive thyroid before sundown. I was not thinking too seriously of the pill's end result, an underactive thyroid. At that point, it did not matter to me. I just wanted the hell of the last ten years to be erased.

Along with my paranoia, I also experienced psychosis. A psychotic paranoid person should not be alone in a hotel room, but I had no choice. When I say I was psychotic, I do not mean Jack-Torrance-in-*The-Shining* psychotic. I would on occasion hear noises, usually whispering, or I would see shadows and find that no one was there. It could have gotten worse, I have no doubt. This mental state forced me to place chairs, a table, an ironing board, you name it, up against the door of that hotel room.

It is unfortunate how underreported most symptoms of a malfunctioning thyroid are. That little pamphlet my endo gave me did not even scratch the surface, which is why I want to tell my story, even if it means revealing my most shameful symptom of them all—yes, worse than the Miracle Ear fiasco. Before I disclose *this* symptom let me just say, I don't judge others for doing what I am about to say, but what I did was not me. It never was before, and it hasn't been since the treatment. You see, as my body began to transform into hyperthyroidism, my libido increased *tremendously*. I was turning into a ninety-year old weakling with extreme joint pain (I could not even open a bottle of water), who had to constantly watch pornography because having multiple orgasms a day was *essential*. There, I said it. Sorry to give you this visual. We are talking going from a very prudish gal to needing sex more than once a day. I even went to a sex toy shop called Peaches and Cream.

It was traumatic for me to enter into this reconverted gingerbread-looking house. This place was, unfortunately, situated on busy thoroughfare. I would have chosen a different place, but it wasn't like I was an authority on where these stores were located. I passed by this one every day on the way to work, so I had an excuse already planned if someone spotted me. "Oh, I thought Peaches and Cream was a place that sold frozen custard." Even the marquee said, "Many lickable flavors to choose from."

I walked into the sex shop toy house with embarrassment, curiosity, and shock all rolled into one. I was shocked at all the different devices I saw—and a little confused. I did not know *where* you were supposed to insert some of the gadgets I saw. I grabbed a couple of items that I recognized, items with er . . . em . . . vibrating features. As I was walking toward the register with my two packages, a man entered who looked like the type of person who would cause you to pull your child close to your hip if he walked by. He nodded to the hotel clerk. Even she threw him an apprehensive nod back. This man walked into a separate section upstairs. A sign was posted at bottom of the staircase: YOU MUST BE 21 TO ENTER. At that point I had seen enough. I didn't even want to know what was up there or see anyone else come in who might want to join that man upstairs. I walked over to the clerk to pay. I wasn't looking around anymore; I just wanted to get out of there. I made no eye contact with anyone. My eyes were fixated on my credit card, ready to hand it to her as soon as I received the amount due. Then the clerk yelled, "Do you need batteries with this?" I was mortified. I wanted to run out as fast as I could. Wow, I never felt that way when the clerk at Toys "R" Us asked me that question. "No," I whispered. I took my purchase and ran out.

Unfortunately, I ended up breaking one of my new toys when I rushed home to boil them in water. After seeing the clientele in that joint, I had felt compelled to sterilize them. Even though they were sealed in vacuum-packed plastic . . . I don't know . . . I thought maybe someone was required to test them out first. My knowledge about this kind of merchandise was pretty much zilch, as evidenced by the glob I turned one of them into during my own sanitizing process. I was left to play with just the *one* working toy because there was no way I was entering that store again. To this day, I still have that sex apparatus, but it is strategically hidden and no doubt collecting dust.

I've touched on many of my symptoms, but oh, there were so many more:

- Continuous watery eyes
- Numbness and tingling in my hands and feet
- Extreme weight loss
- Hair loss
- Diarrhea
- Excessive sweating
- Goiter
- Extreme, constant all-over body pain
- Restless legs
- Muscle atrophy
- Charlie horses nightly
- Dizziness
- Depression
- Stomach pain

- Chronic sinusitis
- Blurred vision. I could not get things into focus most of the time.
- Thoughts of suicide. This was the strangest feeling because I *KNEW* I would never do it, but my mind kept saying over and over again that I wanted to die, that I just *needed* to die. "Carol, you would be better off dead." The sicker I became, the louder this internal grim reaper spoke.
- Extreme memory loss. I cannot remember about 70 percent of my childhood. My mom asked me one day if my childhood memories were gone perhaps because, I had actually been molested by a family friend or a loved one. I laughed at first at her suggestion (I had *not* been abused), but then her statement upset me. My mom knew of my illness. *Why would it be easier for her to accept molestation over a thyroid disease?* I wondered.

It is hard to believe a tiny little gland could cause so much destruction. And yes, despite what medical books, or scientists or anyone else says, the porn and the paranoia were all symptoms just like the aches, pains, and all the other physical issues I had. It is so hard for some to believe that sometimes symptoms from an illness *can* affect someone from the neck up as well as from the neck on down. Thankfully, my extreme sickness—both mental and physical—dissipated after I took that pill.

That radiation-filled pill destroyed that tiny gland so my body would quit attacking itself. The problem with this course of treatment is that it permanently put my body in a state of hypothyroidism. Neither "ism" is fun, but doctors feel hypothyroidism is safer and more manageable than hyperthyroidism. To control hypothyroidism, I must take medication every day for the rest of my life and undergo blood testing every three to six months. The medications are supplements that replace the thyroid hormone that my body is no longer producing naturally. This course of treatment is inconvenient but not horrible. I would rather get a bionic thyroid and become a superhero or something, but since I can't, I will settle for what the used car salesman—err . . . excuse me . . . what the *doctor* sold me: the radioactive pill. Forgive my snark, I feel so much better since RAI treatment. I just wish my endo would have told me all the things the thyroid was in charge of in the body, all the affects of hypothyroidism, and the difficulty I could possibly face trying to get my blood levels within normal range. For example, when I had sinus surgery many years ago, the surgeon explained the brain damage I *could* incur, should his hand happen to slip and shove his surgical instrument up into my cerebral cortex. As horrible as it sounds, I still would like to know these things. I would even take a half-hour, low-budget film about the thyroid made for sixth-grade Health Ed students . . . anything of substance. I hardly call a paltry pamphlet created by the thyroid drug manufacturer an educational tool for someone with thyroid disease. I was in bad shape before RAI, so if the surgeon had fully educated me, it would not have changed my mind; but telling me something valuable would have strengthened her credibility for future visits. I really do not trust most of what she says to me now. I just want my script from her so I can be on my way. When she speaks, I am so tempted to say, "Look, honey, you are just the script giver and nothing else, so get to writing." On the other hand, I should hug her, because the lack of information from her is what drove me to come up with my MacGraver's tips, which I am now sharing with you.

**A promotional message from my MacGraver friend, Susan, who has celiac disease.

It was hard for me to adjust to gluten-free pasta. One day I decided to use chicken broth or beef broth instead of water to cook the pasta. It gave it a much better flavor.

Intermission & Chapter 4 Preview

Nutrition and the Thyroid

As I mentioned before, the thyroid and the brain work closely together.

- The brain requires nutrients and energy.
- The brain uses more energy in the form of glucose and oxygen than any other organ.
- The brain is more dependent on proper energy and metabolism than any other organ.
- The thyroid is largely in control of the energy distributed throughout the body.
- If the thyroid gives off too much or too little energy, this could affect the brain.
- Fruits and vegetables give energy; conversely, processed (junk) foods take it away. Fried food drains energy from all over the body. The average person needs six to eight hours to break down junk food. Someone with an underactive thyroid needs longer.

Foods that can deplete energy

1. Processed sugar
2. Saturated fats
3. Processed flour
4. Alcohol

Foods that can give energy

1. Beans
2. Brown rice
3. Fresh vegetables
4. Fresh fruits

OPTIMAL SERVING SIZES

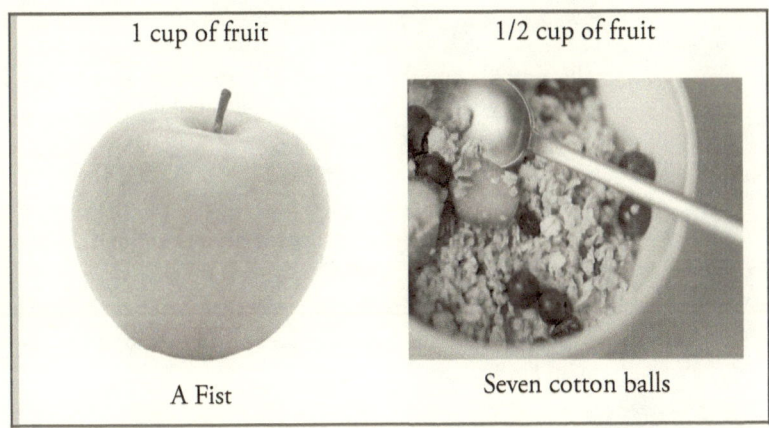

1 cup of fruit

A Fist

1/2 cup of fruit

Seven cotton balls

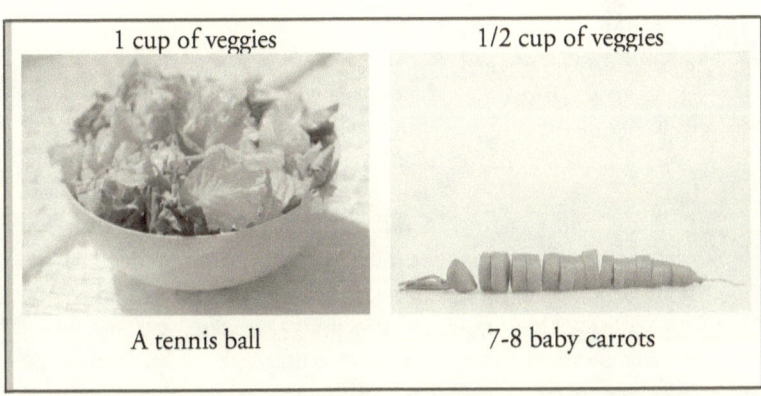

1 cup of veggies

A tennis ball

1/2 cup of veggies

7-8 baby carrots

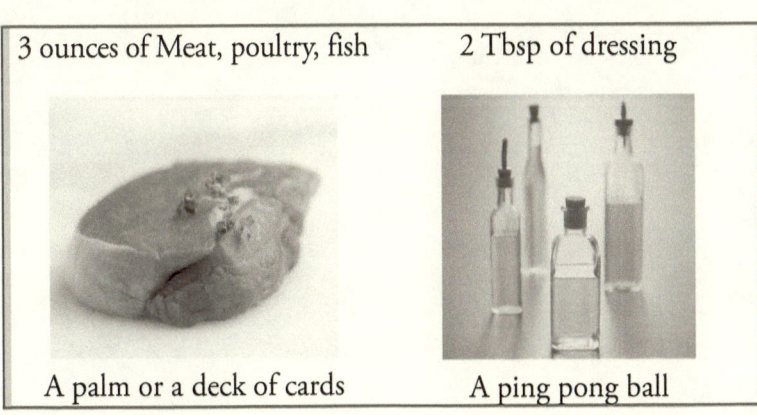

3 ounces of Meat, poultry, fish

A palm or a deck of cards

2 Tbsp of dressing

A ping pong ball

MacGraver's Nutritional Tips

All in the blood: Since your thyroid is no longer working properly and because the thyroid controls metabolism along with the delivery of nutrients to various areas within the body, it is very important to get regular blood work done to gauge hormone, vitamin, and mineral levels. Food sensitivity tests are important as well because digestion troubles. Many doctors won't sign off on regular tests like these; however, you can go to an independent lab and get them done to gauge whether you are within a good range.

Caught on tape: When you are feeling extremely bad, record it! Talk about how you feel, the symptoms, your emotions, and so on. Make a feeling-bad video collection. That way, you can play it back when you are feeling better and you think it is all right to pick up the junk food that had you feeling so bad previously.

Fruits and veggies can put a dent in your wallet: If you have a household like mine—a husband who refuses to eat a fruit or a vegetable and a son who has a limited palate for these kinds of selections—then try getting your produce from the deli. A half cup or a quarter cup of vegetables is less expensive and easier to manage. Buying in small amounts like this can prevent moldy, smelly vegetables in your refrigerator going to waste.

Chapter 4

Nutrition

Months after my radioactive iodine treatment, it had become apparent that I was never going to be the same. This devastating reality was an even harder *pill* to swallow than the one I had taken previously. Growing up in the microwave, fast food, and fax machine era, I had hoped that RAI treatment would, within hours, magically put me back together again. I wanted to be the same *now*. But, I suppose when a God-given appendage is made to become inoperative, a major adjustment is in order. On the bright side, I wasn't exhibiting the extremes that had stricken me before. The paranoid porn-freak zombie had disappeared, thank God! My behavioral about-face makes me wonder about the rest of society. Are the "nut jobs" just a thyroid treatment away from functioning appropriately?

The thyroid medication I take daily helps, but there is no substitute for the real thing. Even though my mental and physical symptoms aren't as severe, it is still apparent when my internal pendulum swings too far hyper or hypo. The difficulties of staying balanced derive from many factors (taking medication on an empty stomach, diet, stress, variations in drug potency with different manufacturers, exposure of the medicine to heat, the list goes on and on). If I focus on these issues too much, I get a headache. Nevertheless, a thyroid sufferer must know his or her body, and constantly be sure not to shift to hyperthyroidism (getting too much thyroid hormone in the body) or hypothyroidism (not getting enough). I had no idea the quest for the middle of the road was going to be a lifelong battle.

Accepting that my old normal was no longer an option, I had to persist with my quest for a new normal, sans a functioning thyroid. And you know, this pursuit has me realizing just how important that tiny butterfly-shaped gland is. Prior to radiation, numerous sage thyroid disease sufferers from social-networking sites suggested I do my research! I took that to mean I should research the various ways to medically treat my condition, which I did. Unfortunately, my research did not encompass the very thing I'd be destroying.

If the thyroid is so darn important, why is destruction or removal the only option for someone with my condition? Again, my imagination started to rev up again. Slipping into my habitual daydreaming mode, I tried to draw a medical parallel to my situation. This is what I came up with:

You are a busy working wife and mother. Toward the end of the school year, your child has a major science project due. This is one of those class assignments requiring mama to trek all over town to various craft, grocery, and art stores for the required class materials. The swifter moms within the county have already seized all the science supplies from the major outlets before you. Consequently, it's taking you an entire week to commandeer all the obscure items needed. As if finding all the goods needed for this project weren't hard enough, you then have to stay on your son or daughter over several weeks to keep them *enthusiastic* about doing it! Cracking the whip on your children is time consuming. Meanwhile, the housework is declining, and other duties are piling up. Your husband has been sick, and his mild cold has inexplicably turned him into a five-year-old. In all the hustle and bustle, you have not given yourself any time for pampering or, at the very least, looking like a human being. You decide to take a bath while giving yourself a mani/pedi.

"Ahhhh." The bath feels good, but suddenly, you look down and notice you have a hangnail on your thumb that is showing signs of an infection. No doubt this is a direct result of neglecting yourself. The next day you call the doctor to see if you can come in for a prescribed topical ointment.

"Sorry, I am unable to give you an ointment. Your finger will have to be amputated."

"What? I don't understand . . ."

"Well, that is what we do with infections to the finger. Just cut that sucker off."

"Isn't there another solution?"

"Nope. But what I *can* do is whittle one of my tongue depressors into the shape of a thumb, and voila! A replacement!"

Okay, so this illustration is a little inane, but you get my point. Why the extreme medical treatment? Why not a thyroid transplant? Why not input bionic parts or try to understand *why* the gland goes haywire, so that it can possibly be restored back to functional? Is removal or destruction the *best* choice for patients?

So let's see . . . They destroyed a vital part of me, and then prescribed pills as a "replacement" for that all too-important gland. Geesh, so why in the world did I think I would ever be the same again? Don't get me wrong: I am not kicking myself for taking the radioactive pill. I am just frustrated at the choices (or lack thereof) given to patients in the twenty-first century.

Then, out of the blue, a wave of compassion befell me, like what the Grinch suddenly felt for the dwellers of Whoville. Maybe the medical community has no idea how critical the thyroid gland is to the human body. I mean, that pamphlet given to me by the endo touched on it briefly, but it wasn't *60 Minutes*-type coverage.

During a recent gynecological exam, an older doctor within my OB-GYN practice, who had not examined me before, was kind enough to describe in great detail how my uterus was tilted too far back toward my pelvis. He went onto say that in medical school his generation had been taught that women with this condition would never be able to have children. He said that he and his colleagues had given this incorrect information out for many years. I dolefully snickered because I remember being told that news by several doctors over a span of a few years when I was younger. Luckily, my hardheaded, stubborn teenager mentality allowed this grim news to go in one ear and out the other. I knew if God wanted me to have children, I would have them. My uterus could have been lodged in my elbow—it did not matter. But sadly, countless babies did not make their arrival into this world, or perhaps some were conceived unintentionally, because of this medical misinformation.

Thus, for a span of several decades or maybe longer, childbearing women were given poor medical advice. Surely there had to have been one or two patients with an off-kilter uterus who had given birth right in front of a doc's eyes. Did these Masters of Medicine feel it was unimportant to spread the word promptly? I mean, they had just delivered what must have seemed to be a miraculous bundle of joy. Couldn't one or two of them have said, "Ummm . . . Hey, guys . . . We were, like, unfortunately taught the wrong thing"? Giving them the benefit of the doubt, maybe they did tell others and news in this community just travels slowly. Nevertheless, here's the bottom line: the thyroid gland is vital, and if it isn't functioning properly, your body becomes a dysfunctional family of the worst kind. Medical professionals need to understand what goes wrong in our bodies sooner, rather than later. We cannot wait decades for this kind of news to get to them. If I have to pull out the heavy artillery (my gossiping neighbor) to spread the word, well, then that's what I'll do!

In the meantime, I am still fine-tuning my MacGraver's tricks to muddle through. In fact, a few years after my RAI treatment, as I adjusted to my new normal, nothing could touch me. My stress-coping tricks were working like a charm; I deflected those stress weights like I was wearing a pair of Wonder Woman's wrist thingies. But then I received a major blow that brought me to my knees: my father's cancer diagnosis, which lead to his eventual passing. The cancer consumed his body, spreading from his prostate to his bones and then to his brain. His deterioration came on suddenly. He was here, and then—*poof!*—he was gone; at least, that is how it seemed. My family's first major loss heavily impacted us all; it was almost unbearable. The anguish penetrated an armor I had constructed for myself to keep away other autoimmune diseases and bacterial and viral infections. However, this was beyond stress. Stress would have been too afraid to go near this territory. So what happened as a result? I became sick for about four months. I went to work (barely) each weekday morning, and then I came home. That's about it! On the weekends, I spent most of my time convalescing in bed. That is when I began penning this book. My brain was motivated, just not the rest of me. Autoimmune disease sufferers know that illnesses come quite frequently and tend to linger longer than with the average person. You hate this, I know. Me too!

After my father's death, I had ailments the likes of which my body had never seen. The worst sore throat of my life, swollen glands in every bodily area that housed glands, blisters on the inside and outside of my mouth, and daily headaches. A fever did not accompany this malaise, though, which had me fearing another autoimmune disorder.

Death is inevitable, and so are other hardships I cannot control. I had mastered the standard stressors in life, but how could I work on keeping my body healthy after something serious, like a loved one's death? I initially thought I had been handling my father's death well; regular visits to a therapist and leaning on my family for support were great coping methods. But there was one dear old friend I paid too much attention to during this time. I had sought help from this friend before to get me through difficult situations, perhaps overusing this pal of mine. No, it wasn't alcohol this time; I was done with that. My *extreme* anxiety had dissipated, so there was no need for me to drink anymore. This was another self-soother: junk food. I comforted myself with various sugary goodies, fried foods, and the worst carbs sold east of the Mississippi.

The more I shoveled down poor nutritional provisions, the sicker I became. Two rounds of antibiotics, three doctor appointments, and an ER visit didn't help. I also might not have been helping myself by taking those numerous prescribed antibiotics; they might have been killing the good bacteria as well as the bad. Fed up and frustrated, I decided to eat nothing but fresh fruits and vegetables for two days. For the first time in what seemed like forever, I started to feel well enough to walk around with the living again.

To a thyroid autoimmune disease sufferer, a moment of feeling fantastic is like winning the lottery. My newfound healthy fortune had me wondering why two days of eating nothing but fruits and veggies had broken my four-month infirmity. (Time to go back to Google! If all of my various MDs knew of my Googling behavior, they would most certainly superglue my hands together.)

Various articles, health websites, and archived medical abstracts, helped me understand how and why infections seem to stick around the body of a chronically ill individual. Again, in my own *simplistic* way, I've deduced why I became so sick and, more important, why I stayed sick for so long:

- My autoimmune disease + My thyroid disease = Chronic infections

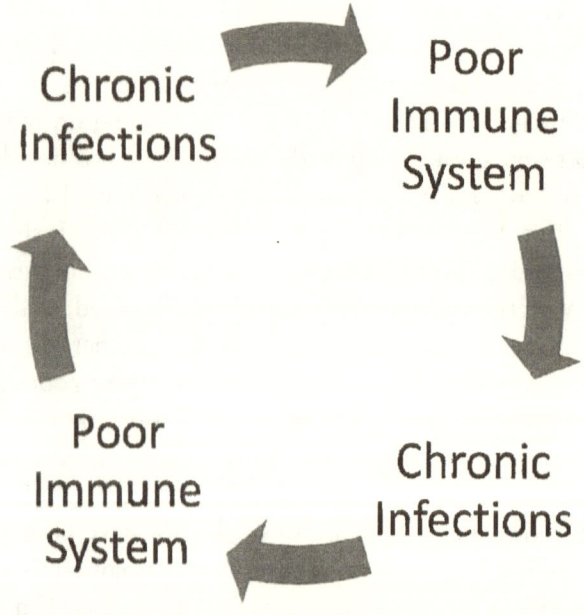

- Chronic infections = Poor immune system
- Poor immune system = Chronic infections

I really want off this vicious immune system cycle. I sought after medical doctors who specialize in autoimmunity, attempting to reach them directly by telephone. No luck. An immunologist (without the "auto") was the closest, but these doctors are primarily allergists (at least in my state). I know this because I called every one of them to see if there was hope for an autoimmune-disease sufferer like myself, but no such luck. After perusing the directory of specialists I noticed that the majority of the bodily systems were covered:

- Nervous system (Neurologist)
- Cardiovascular system (Cardiologist)
- Endocrine system (Endocrinologist)
- Musculoskeletal system (Orthopedist or Rheumatologist)
- Digestive system (Gastroenterologist)
- Respiratory system (Pulmonologist)
- Reproductive system (Gynecologist)

If I break my leg or if the old ticker is acting screwy, there's no question which doc I would need to see. But where do I go for an autoimmune disease? I've talked to so many autoimmune-disease sufferers who have been treated by herbalists, gynecologists, rheumatologists, homeopaths, apothecaries, and their local psychics for their autoimmune diseases. Does anyone else feel like something is wrong with this picture? If I told someone I was going to the gynecologist for my heart, they would probably give me a tongue lashing, warning about how unsafe that is. But it is okay to go to that same gyno for an autoimmune disease? Some might argue that a heart problem could potentially be fatal and should be taken more seriously. And I would say that an autoimmune disease poses the same risk. *Autoimmune* means your body is attacking itself, and since you only have one body, it is kind of important to find a way to stop it from doing that. There may be much that is still not known about the immune system; it is somewhat foreign to the medical community. Scientists are constantly discovering new information about our solar system. Perhaps there is still more to know about the systems within our body.

Eventually, it was time for more Googling. I began researching the location of the immune system within the human body. Mine absolutely hates my guts, so I should know where my enemy hangs out, right? It turns out the majority of the immune system works predominately *in the gut.*

- Depending on what source you read, 60 to 80 percent of your immune system dwells within your digestive system.
- Your digestive system is comprised of your
  a. Mouth
  b. Esophagus
  c. Liver
  d. Stomach
  e. Gallbladder
  f. Pancreas
  g. Large intestine
  h. Small intestine
  i. Appendix
  j. Rectum
  k. Anus

Thinking back to all the digestive tract disorders I have had over the years leading up to my autoimmune disease (gall bladder issues, irritable bowel syndrome, esophagitis, mouth sores, spastic colon, fissure), I wonder if this could have been a precursor to my Graves' disease diagnosis? Was my body trying to warn me, screaming at me, "EAT BETTER OR ELSE!" Shoving garbage into the central location of your immune system is not going to keep you well—trust me—especially if, out of the gate, you are already in poor health. My gastrointestinal issues significantly decreased after I made the decision to drastically cut back on gluten. I believe we thyroidians have a hard time digesting even the simplest of foods. So, when you add a genetically altered pasta dish with more gluten than what was intended for us to consume, it can cause a whole slew of GI difficulties. For more info about our genetically altered wheat products, see: http://enhanced-life.blogspot.com/2011/11/so-what-big-deal-about-gluten.html.

—

MacGraver's Tip

Remember, comfort food isn't so comforting when your body starts an uprising. It may not be verbal communication, but your body will certainly tell you when it needs something nutritious. Listen to it!

—

Why did food become so complicated and the object of such great indulgence? There must be something to those clichéd maxims: "You are what you eat." "Your body is like a car; it needs the proper fuel to run efficiently." I have heard many a doctor give that car analogy. Yawn! This parallel was always lost on me because it lacked the necessary theatrics to get my attention. I'm sure this illustration is effective with males, but to get my attention, docs need to paint vivid, sometimes graphic, pictures. For example: "Cars need to be washed and given the proper fuel, and they need those all-too-important regular oil changes. If you fail do those things for your car, it will break down, possibly when it is 100 degrees outside or 20 degrees below zero and you are on the highway, heading to work for a very important meeting." Adversity or painting the picture of adversity breeds common sense, at least for moi. If you can tell me the why, what, when, and how, you have my undivided attention. *Why* does the car need fuel, *what* will happen if I do not supply it, and *when* and *how* will it break down? "Your body is like a car, and it needs the proper fuel" is a vague robotic statement. It may sound reasonable, but why would I trust this statement if I have no frame of reference as to the repercussions of improper fuel. To test my theory of how we are told what to do, but not given information about why, I asked several people, "When you were in school, what were you told about food?" The majority of them said, "That we are supposed to eat a balanced diet from the food pyramid."

"Why?" I asked.

"Because it is good for you," they replied.

"Why is it good for you?"

"It just is. It makes you healthy."

"Okay, what does healthy look like?"

Blank looks and shrugged shoulders.

Could this be why our diets in this country get progressively worse year after year? We do not receive enough education on what poor eating can do to the body. The Centers for Disease Control and Prevention reported on a near ten-year study on fruit and vegetable consumption within the United States. This study revealed, shockingly, that none of our states met the target goal.[1] Not one state! In fact, our produce intake seems to be decreasing each year. Could that explain the increasing number of diseases in America? For a developed country with the knowledge and the distribution channels at our disposal, our disease dossier does not look good.

Remember those Sally Struthers commercials on late-night television asking us to help feed starving children in Africa. If you're like me, you might have tried to turn the channel quickly. I never wanted to see what malnutrition or poor nutrition could do to a person, but maybe I should have. Poor eating is serious, and although the situation

---

[1] Centers for Disease Control, State-Specific Trends and Vegetable Consumption Amoung Adults—United States, September 10, 2010, accessed July 20, 2011, http://www.cdc.gov/mmwr/preview/mmwrhtml/mm5935a1.htm.

in parts of Africa and elsewhere in the world is extreme, Americans may not be too far behind in the international poor diet race.

Our country needs to quit focusing on what we should eat and start educating us on what will happen if we *don't* eat nutritionally. Describe *in detail* how diabetes can systematically eat away at the body and what obesity can do to the heart. And thyroid sufferer, I'm sure you have a compelling story. Although, I cannot say 100 percent for sure that poor nutrition was the root cause of my four-month hiatus, I do know that, while my dad was dying (and even after his death), I never grabbed carrot sticks or apples as my comfort food.

After I had exhausted all other medical avenues, my two-day fruit and vegetable medicinal body makeover had me well again; and now that I know where my immune system is located, MacGraver has a plan! I am going to incorporate more nutritional foods into my diet, whether I am feeling well or not. I absolutely love to cook. I have several friends who don't and are constantly asking me how I prepare certain dishes. Below I have included a grid and pictures that show the various ways to prepare vegetables. I've also included a list of fruits as well.

VEGETABLES

Fresh	Raw, wash them off and you are ready to eat as is
Steam	Microwave steaming-Use a microwave safe dish, place the veggies in. Add a very small amount of water, cover (not completely) cook for 3-6 minutes depending on taste and the vegetable.
Grill	Place your favorite veggies on the grill, season and cook to taste.
Bake or Broil	Put your favorite vegetable on a baking or broiler pan and place in the oven. There are many recipes in books and on the internet advising on the favorable cooking times and temperatures.
Sauté	Use a skillet good for sautéing, add olive oil or butter. Season to taste.

FRESH

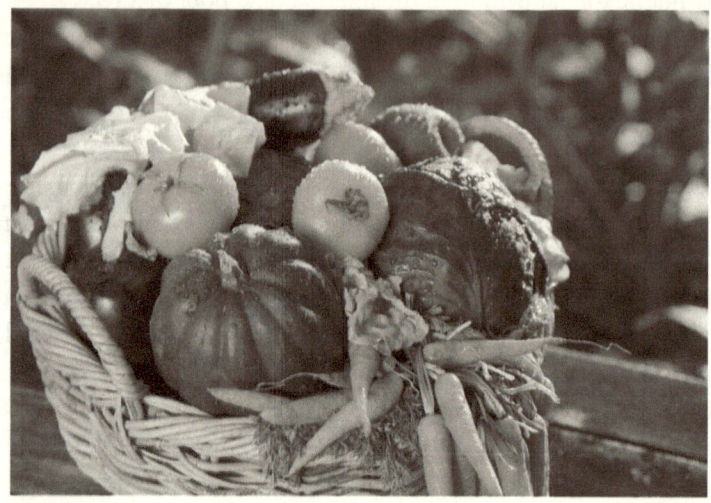

Peppers I like to buy red, yellow, and green peppers, slice them and eat them raw.

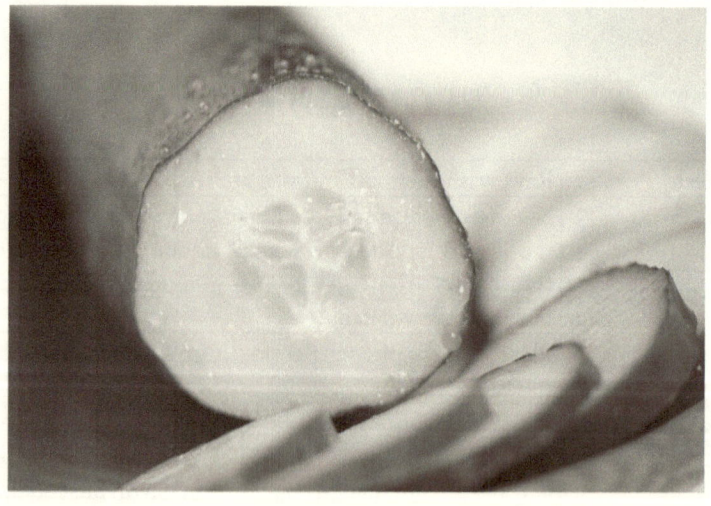

Cucumbers Drizzle with an oil-and-vinegar dressing. Yum.

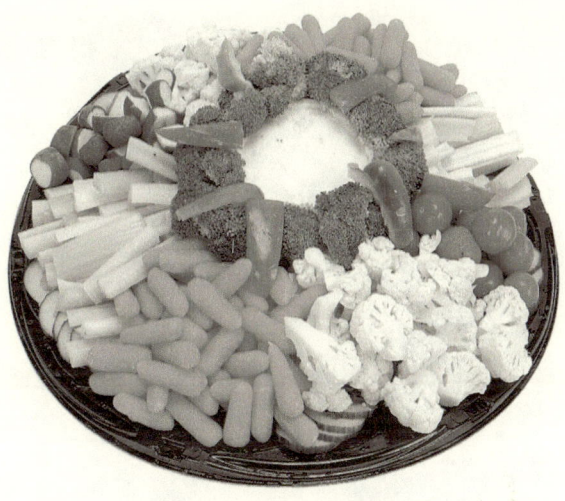

Veggie tray Purchase one at your local grocery store. You and the family can munch for a week or two, or take some out for a salad.

SAUTÉED

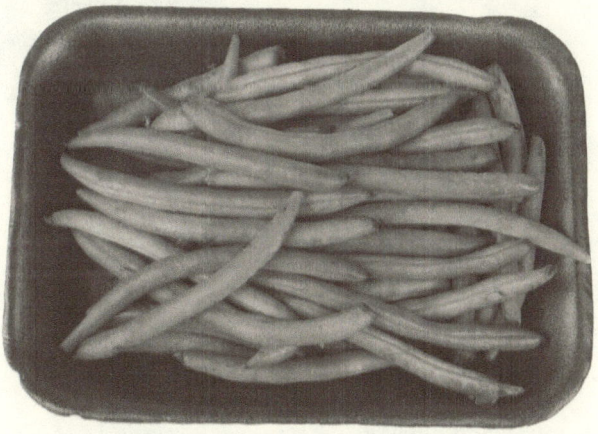

Green beans I purchase these fresh in the produce section and then sauté them with garlic and olive oil for about five minutes.

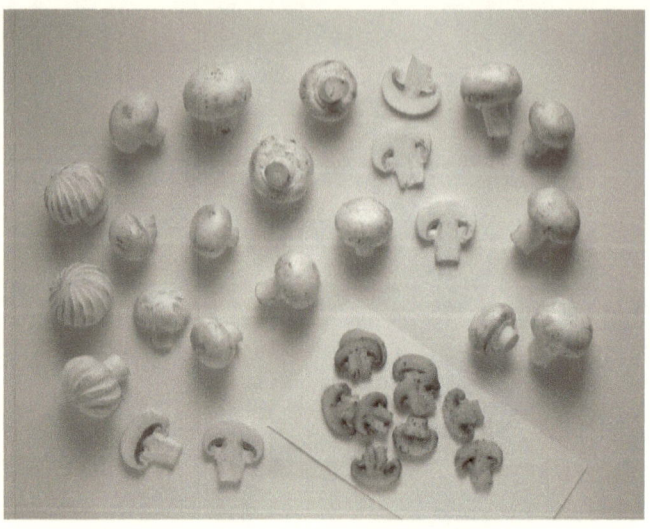

Mushrooms These taste great sautéed with other vegetables or by themselves with just a little butter and salt and pepper.

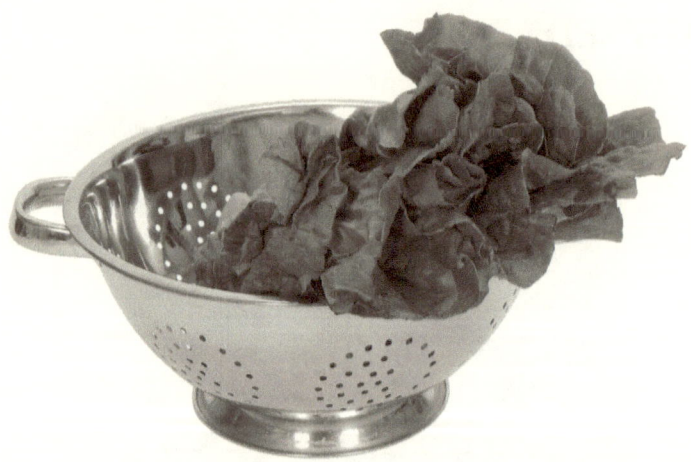

Spinach Sauté, add olive oil, sesame seeds, salt and pepper to make this delish dish!

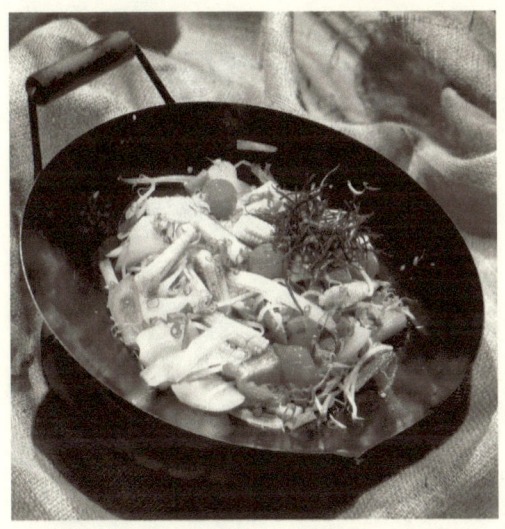

Throw everything in Add chicken or shrimp, and you have a nice stir-fry!

STEAM

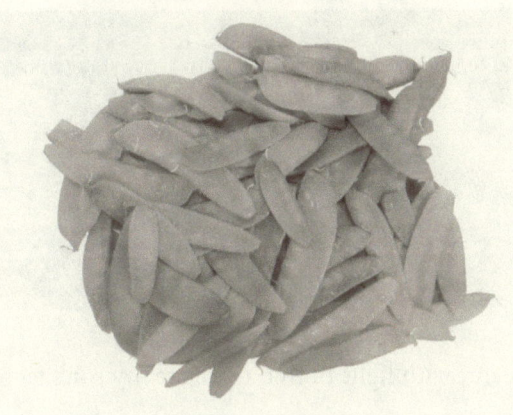

Snow peas Steam your snow peas with salt and pepper or Asian seasoning.

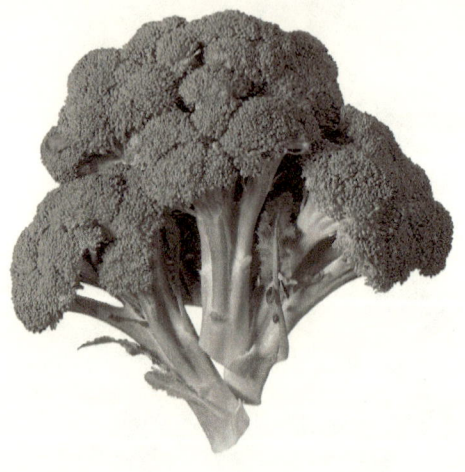

Broccoli If the only way you can eat steamed broccoli is with cheese, add just a small amount.

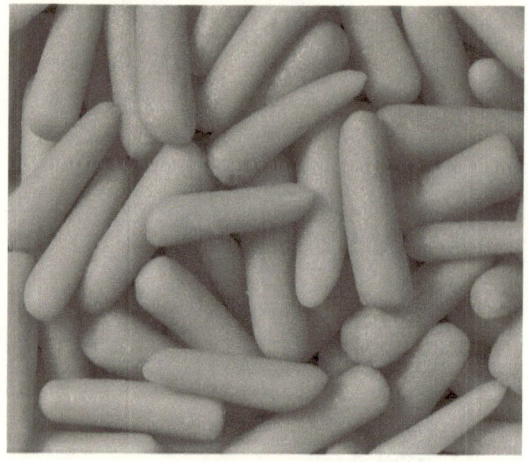

Carrots Steam, with light butter, these are my son's favorite.

BAKED

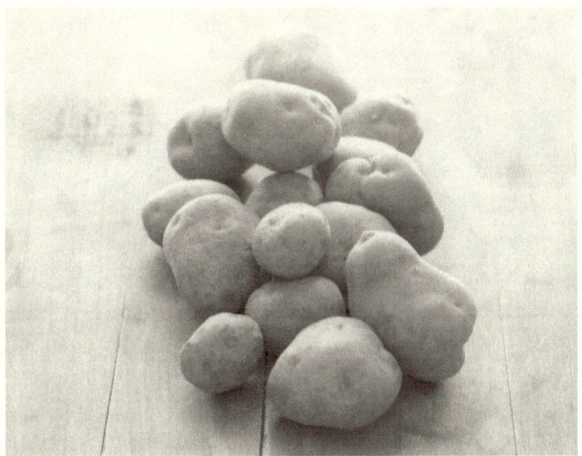

Potato Go easy on the butter and sour cream if that's the only way you can eat a baked potato. Or you might want to try healthy toppings like homemade salsa.

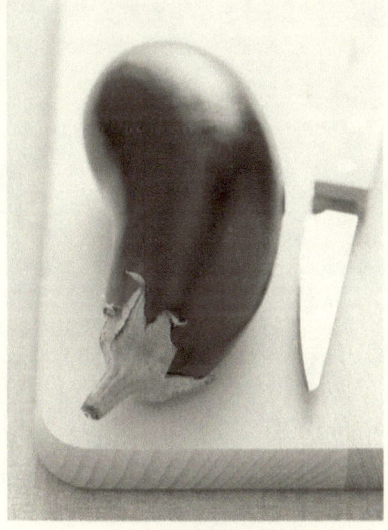

Eggplant The only way I can eat eggplant is by making eggplant parmesan. Many delicious recipes can be found on the internet.

GRILLED

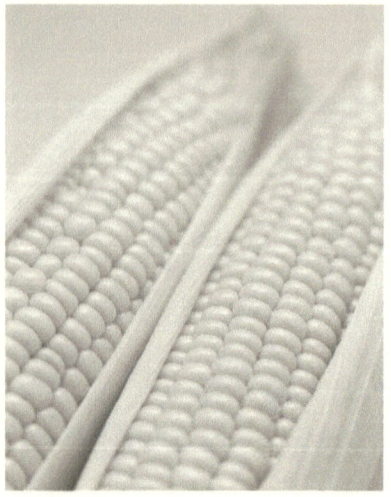

Corn on the cob I typically like to grill my corn on the cob, that way I don't have to put tons of butter on it. The grill gives it so much flavor that all I need is a little salt and pepper.

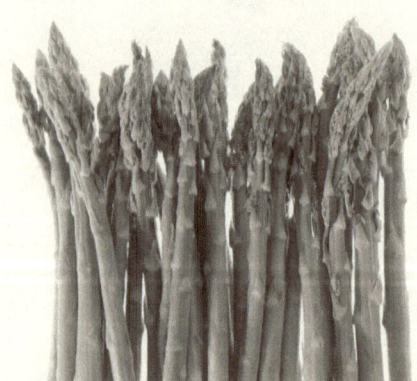

Asparagus These veggies are very good sprinkled with olive oil and seasoning.

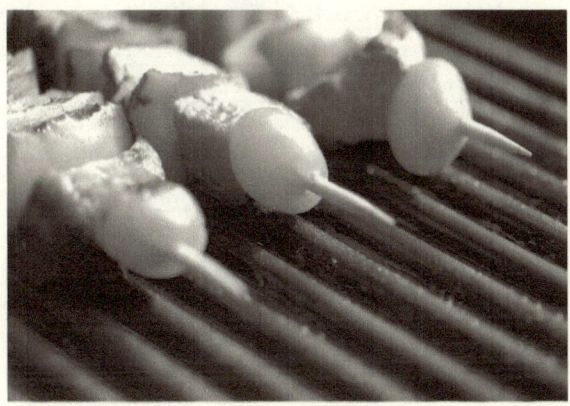

Tomatoes Tomatoes aren't my favorite, but I don't mind them grilled. Grilled tomatoes in a salad give it great flavor.

VEGETABLE'S NUTRITIONAL VALUE

Type	Benefits	Best in
Garlic	B6, C, Manganese, Calcium, Copper	Aug-Oct
Leeks	Fiber, Folic Acid	Sep-March
Onions	Chromium, Biotin	Aug-Oct
Scallions	Chromium, Biotin	Year-round
Shallots	Chromium, Biotin	Jun-Aug
Cucumbers	Vitamin K, Potassium,	May-Sep
Eggplant	B-Complex,	May-Aug
Zucchini	Vitamin A, C	May-Aug
Peppers	Vitamin A, C, Magnesium and Selenium	May-Oct
Squash	Vitamin A, B-Complex, Riboflavin	May-Aug
Tomatoes	Vitamin A, C, Folic Acid	May-Oct
Artichokes	Iron, Iodine, Vitamin A and C	Mar-June
Broccoli	Vitamin A and C, Folic Acid	Nov-Mar
Cauliflower	Fiber, B-6	Jan-Dec
Brussels Sprouts	Fiber, and Vitamin C	Sep-Mar
Cabbage	Vitamin B5, B6, K, Fiber, Folic Acid	Jan-Dec
Collards	Vitamin C and K, Lutein, Folates	Sep-Mar

Lettuce	Vitamin A, Beta-Carotene, Zeaxanthin	Jun-Sep
Spinach	Vitamin A, C, Iron, Potassium, Beta-Carotene	May-Oct
Beets	Vitamin C, Folates, Fiber, Flavonoid	Jun-Feb
Carrots	Vitamin A, C, Beta-Carotene, Copper,	Jul-Mar
Radishes	Vitamin B-6, Riboflavin, Thiamin, Iron	May-Oct
Turnip	Vitamin A, B-Complex, C and K	Jun-Jan
Potato	Starch, B-complex, Iron, Manganese, Copper	Jun-Jul
Asparagus	Vitamin A, C, E, Iron, Riboflavin	May-Jun
Celery	Vitamin C	Jul-Nov
Fennel	Vitamin C, Anethole, Selenium, Zinc	Jul-Oct

FRUITS

FRUIT	NUTRITIONAL VALUES IN ORDER (health concerns)
Apples	flavonoids, fiber, C (pesticides, wax coating)
Apricots	carotenoids, A, C, fiber (preservatives)
Bananas	B6, C, potassium (glycemic)
Blackberries	flavonoids, fiber, C, K, manganese
Blueberries	flavonoids, C, manganese, fiber
Cantaloupe	carotenoids, C, A, potassium
Cherries	flavonoids (pesticides)
Cranberries	flavonoids, fiber, C, manganese
Dates	(glycemic)
Dried fruit	(glycemic, preservatives)
Figs	(preservatives)
Fruit juices	(glycemic)
Grapefruit	carotenoids in pink, flavonoids, C
Grapes	flavonoids, manganese (pesticides)
Guava	carotenoids, fiber, C
Kiwifruit	C, fiber (glycemic)
Lemons	flavonoids, C (wax coating)
Limes	flavonoids, C (wax coating)
Mangoes	carotenoids, A, C (glycemic)
Nectarines	carotenoids, C (glycemic, pesticides)
Oranges	carotenoids, flavonoids, C, fiber (glycemic)

Papayas	carotenoids, C, folate, potassium
Peaches	carotenoids, C (pesticides)
Pears	flavonoids (pesticides)
Persimmons	C (glycemic)
Pineapple	C, manganese (glycemic)
Plums	carotenoids, C
Raspberries	flavonoids, fiber, manganese, C
Raisins	(glycemic, pesticides, preservatives)
Strawberries	carotenoids, flavonoids, C, fiber (pesticides)
Tangerines	carotenoids, A, C (glycemic)
Watermelon	carotenoids, C, A, B6 (glycemic)

This is not an exhaustive list of fruits because I primarily want to focus on the common produce readily available in stores. Also, certain items are only indigenous to a geographical area.

RECOMMENDED DAILY ALLOWANCE OF VITAMINS AND MINERALS

Nutrient	RDA
Vitamin A	900 µg
Vitamin C	60 mg
Calcium	1000 mg
Iron	18 mg
Vitamin D	400 IU (10 µg)
Vitamin E	30 IU
Vitamin K	80 µg
Thiamin	1.5 mg
Riboflavin	1.7 mg
Niacin	20 mg
Vitamin B6	2 mg
Folate	400 µg
Vitamin B12	6 µg
Biotin	300 µg
Pantothenic acid	10 mg

Phosphorus	1000 mg
Iodine	150 µg
Magnesium	400 mg
Zinc	15 mg
Selenium	70 µg
Copper	2 mg
Manganese	2 mg
Chromium	120 µg
Molybdenum	75 µg
Chloride	3400 mg

µg = Microgram
IU = International unit
mg = Milligram

—

My MacGraver's arsenal is looking better and better. I never again want to resemble Charlie's grandparents from Willy Wonka (bedridden). I mean, this is about survival. I know I keep saying that, but it is true. If you were stranded on a desert island, you would find a way to survive. Survival techniques would be essential on that island. You wouldn't say, "I am not eating this fish I caught because it lacks a creamy béarnaise sauce."

My memory is shot all to hell, which is why I am continuously baffled by the random information that is stored in my memory bank and by what later gets deposited in the forefront of my mind. For example, I used to watch the reality television show *Survivor* in which contestants are stuck in a remote location and must survive on a limited amount of food. In the second season, Tina Wesson won the million-dollar prize, and as the time of my writing this, she holds the record for being the oldest female *Survivor* winner. I will never forget how, during an interview after her win, she revealed that she suffered from a debilitating autoimmune condition called rheumatoid arthritis. She said the severe aches and pains that go along with RA were nonexistent throughout her time on the show in a remote area of Australia. Tina, a nurse, firmly believes her diet of primarily fruits, veggies, and fish was the reason for the diminished signs of her disease. I was not familiar with autoimmune diseases at that time, so seeing her discuss her autoimmune disease did not mean much to me then. Perhaps this wasn't technically a memory, but my angel screaming at me, "HEY, YOU HEARD TINA'S TESTIMONY FOR A REASON!"

Okay, so I've established what stress and a lack of nutrition can do. Gone are the days when I could gluttonously gratify myself with any kind of food I want. Well, at least I had a good forty-plus-year run. But now I am waving the white flag. You win, body. I will now feed you things you can work with. I want you to say, "Ahhh, yes, I can do great things with this little morsel. I will give it to this cell . . . oh, and that one over there." I will get my body to love me again, even if it kills me.

**I interrupt this program to bring you one of my MacGraver friends, Nikki, who lives with fibromyalgia.

If we only listen to our bodies, we all would do better. I believe in the raw food movement, this is what has mainly worked for me. I drink lots a water daily and juice whenever I can. It took me a year, but determination is a strong force. The entire system worked for me without major investments other than buying good food and eating it, even if I didn't want it.

I don't believe a real cure lies within conventional medicine, and we need to open our eyes to take charge of our own health. Expecting medical doctors to take us seriously could take a lifetime.

Chapter 4

The Sequel

What do Kim Catrall, Jillian Michaels, Kim Alexis, and Mary-Louise Parker have in common? They all have hypothyroidism. I know what you are thinking: So why aren't these gals being rolled down the red carpet like Violet Beauregarde in *Willy Wonka and the Chocolate Factory*? Instead, they are svelte, sexy women—with *hypothyroidism*! Oprah comes to mind as the only famous plus-size gal who is hypo. Perhaps it's because our girl Oprah's livelihood is not contingent upon whether or not she can fit into Barbie-doll clothing. Her millions—pardon me, her billions—were made by sitting on a couch each week. We love and accept Oprah just as she is, nice and plump. I am not sure if the aforementioned Hollywood honeys would have quite the same level of success with Oprah's junk in the trunk. Sad reality, but true. Most of the celeb elite maintain the toned physiques that are pretty much a requirement in order to remain on the Hollywood hilltops. Wanting to stay there is, of course, a huge incentive for them to stay lean. I am heavier now because of my hypothyroidism, but what is *my* motivation to become lean?

Unfortunately we live in a society where being lean is equated with being healthy and beautiful—the epitome of which is the Hollywood bombshell. So, many of us strive for the toned Hollywood body, seeking healthy and not-so-healthy methods to get there—myself included. When I gained a lot of weight after radioactive iodine treatment, "depressed" would not even begin to describe how I felt. I became mortified because this was a new thing for me. Anyway I could, I tried to lose the weight I had suddenly gained, mostly using those not-so-healthy methods. Nothing worked.

My subconscious was telling me that if I got back to my old weight, all would be right again. I would be healthy, I would feel good, and of course, I would be happy. But then it dawned on me that prior to my diagnosis, I *was* thin—and also very sick. So thin does not necessarily mean healthy or happy. Lightbulb moment: If my sole focus is to get thin instead of healthy, than I will not be successful. I suddenly heard a *Field of Dreams* whisper: "Carol, go for healthy, and thin will come."

If you could not already tell by now, I am the type of gal who needs to know why. As I was growing up, "why" was constantly coming out of my mouth when my parents asked me to do things. "Why do I need to clean my room?" "Why do I need to go to school?" "Why I can't watch that television show?" If the reason was good enough, I would go with it; if not, then I would not cooperate, or if I did, it would be with great reluctance. This brings me to my biggest question: How do I get healthy? It sure as heck ain't gonna come by getting a TSH test every three months and taking T3 and T4 meds. I've done this for more than five years now. My MacGraver's tricks stabilize me, but I want more—I want to feel great.

I don't care about fitting into the latest clothing line, impressing my husband, or living to be one hundred. I have a chronic disease. I am a wife, a mother, and an employee. I need to function successfully, and in order to do this I need to eat nutritionally and exercise. This is my motivation! Oh, and also to drastically reduce those doctor bills. A slender physique will come as a result. Doing something for the *right* reasons will reap better results in the end.

After my moment of clarity, I made an appointment with a dietician right away. She put me on the following 1,200-calorie diet:

CALORIES PER DAY

	1200	1600	1800	2000	2200
Starches	75 gm	105 gm	120 gm	135 gm	150 gm
Fruits	45 gm	45 gm	45 gm	60 gm	60 gm
Milk	45 gm	45 gm	45 gm	45 gm	45 gm
Sweets/Deserts Other Carbo-hydrates					
Nonstarchy Vegetables	15 gm	60 gm	75 gm	90 gm	90 gm
Meat & Meat Substitutes	4 oz	6 oz	6 oz	7 oz	9 oz

I was able to get as far as three days on this diet, and then I quit. A few weeks later I tried again for a week and then quit again. A couple of months passed, and I decided to give it a go one more time. And then—yes, that's right—I quit. Finally, I realized I could not follow the dietician's meal plan in the state I was in. You see, I've always had trouble with consistent nutrition and exercise when I feel like crap. Physically, years after my diagnosis, I had more bad days than good. Autoimmune disease flare-ups are a kind of a hell on earth. When I felt bad, exercise was out of the question, and when it came to meals, grabbing the quickest, easiest morsels (which was usually the *least* nutritious) was all I was capable of doing. Cutting up vegetables for a nice healthy salad sounds easy enough, but for the chronically ill, the thought of accomplishing a task even this size is nearly impossible. I needed to cleanse/detox my body before I could attempt any dietary plan. I needed to heal on the inside. Some experts say it is always good to cleanse your body before beginning a nutritious dietary program. This process will rid the body of toxins, making it easier for the fat to burn. For more info on this see the article, "How to Cleanse Your Body before Dieting," found here: http://www.livestrong.com/article/107334-cleanse-body-before-dieting/.

I remembered back when I had done that two-day fruit-and-vegetable diet after becoming nearly bedridden following my dad's death. I decided this time to do a ten-day cleanse that I sort of made up. I had tried juicing previously, but I believe having a bum thyroid may not be conducive to that sort of program. I became very sick with blood sugar issues while doing the juicing, so I came up with my own detoxing plan as an alternative.

This is what I did:

Days 1-5

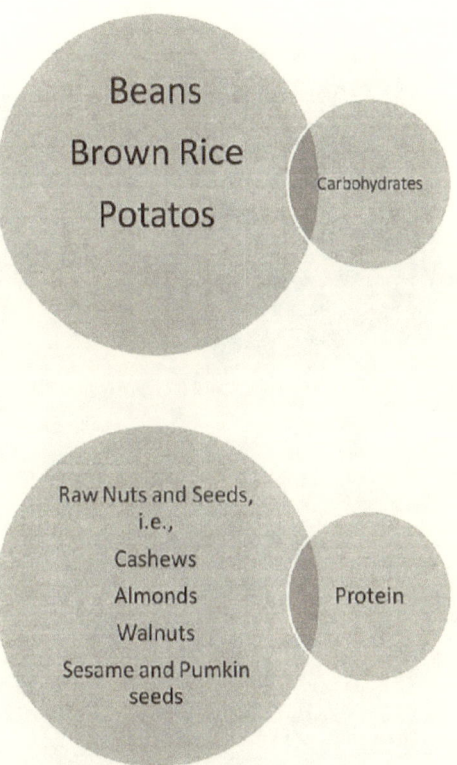

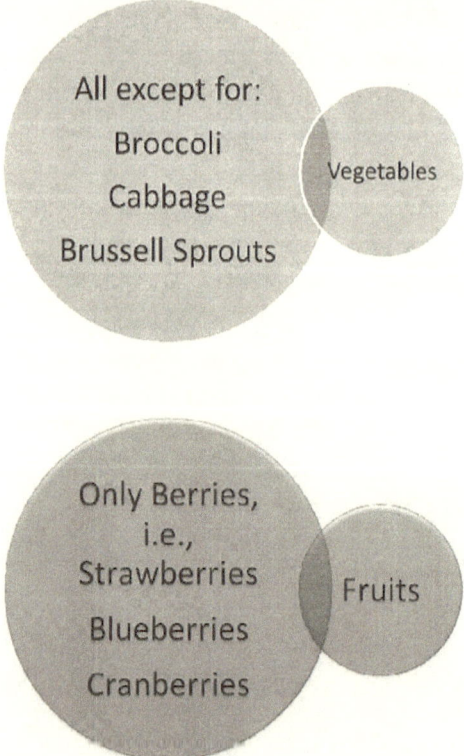

All except for:
Broccoli
Cabbage
Brussell Sprouts

Vegetables

Only Berries,
i.e.,
Strawberries
Blueberries
Cranberries

Fruits

Days 5-10

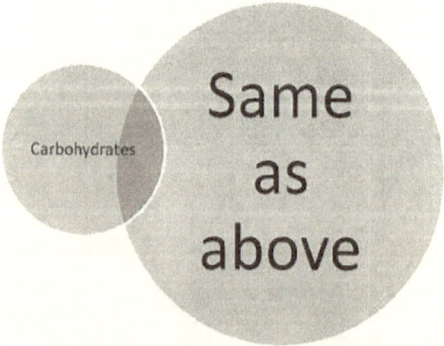

Carbohydrates

Same
as
above

Protein

Same as above plus add fish, baked or grilled not fried

Vegetables

Same as above plus add all other vegetables

Fruit

Same as above plus add all fruit

Day 1: Wednesday

The day starts out okay. I've done cleanses before (before my thyroid disease), and day one usually consists of a few hunger pangs sprinkled throughout the day. This is why it is always important to have a lot of food and water on hand that first day.

I am not sure if cleansing your body when it is diseased makes a difference, but day one is quite different this time around. A headache comes on around midday. In the past, the junk-food-withdrawal headache usually occurred on day two or three; so based on my previous experiences, I decided to go to my job on the first day of cleansing. Big mistake.

The headache intensifies with each hour. The workday begins to slow down, and my withdrawal symptoms speed up. Extreme nausea comes on, followed by dizziness and sweating. This withdrawal is ugly, almost like something you would expect to see with a crack addict. I sneak out of work a half hour early; I cannot take it anymore. I have to quickly get supine or I'll be hugging the toilet bowl—hardly the condition one should be in at the workplace. I get home and spend about an hour dry-heaving over the toilet. Then I take two melatonin pills. I'm out for the evening.

Day 2: Thursday

I am *very close* to giving up, but then I remember why I started all this in the first place. One day of feeling like I have the worst hangover of my life will be a small price to pay for this detoxification. Hopefully, the worst of it is over.

Crankiness is my only setback on day two; I get into it with my manager and the chief operating officer. Note to self: next time take a few days off during the initial cleansing process.

Day 3: Friday

The crankiness runneth over . . . but now I am having clear and concise thoughts. My communication skills are elevated, and my cranky tongue has never been more intellectual. The biggest plus? I have enough energy to go out with friends after work. This is not the norm for me. Friday fatigue gets the best of me more often than not.

Day 4: Saturday

I've lost five pounds! So nothing else matters. Kidding aside, this weight was mainly water, I'm sure. Usually on day four of my other cleanses, I turn the corner and feel great. I am not feeling great, but I do feel good. I am hoping great will come soon.

Day 5: Sunday

The true test! I dutifully go to my sister-in-law's birthday party at a nice restaurant. I know going in that the meal will be free. This means I can have my choice of a delicious fruity cocktail, a high-caloric entrée, and a rich, sinful desert. The other five people at the table do just that, but I am happy to report that I have a Mediterranean salad with vinaigrette dressing and without the feta cheese. When it comes to food, will power is not my strong suit, but this time I manage to do it! I feel good today, still not great, but I am hopeful. I will get there soon.

Day 6: Monday

I am spending a lot of time on the toilet. This is a good thing, right? I mean, isn't this what cleansing is all about?

Day 7: Tuesday

Okay, my poop is really, *really* grossing me out. If your feces is supposed to give any indication of your health, then I am scared. I am tempted to scoop it out with a fishing net and take it to the nearest hospital lab. It has white, creepy, swirly things in it . . . Back to Google.

Day 8: Wednesday

I Googled my poop, and I HAVE WORMS! I meet all the criteria for symptoms, and these suckers are coming out in droves each time I go to the bathroom. Sorry for this graphic picture, but I feel it is important to talk to my autoimmune family about this sensitive topic. You see, parasitic worms are very common; we all have them. A normal immune system will continuously flush them out, but they will flourish in sick bodies. Not only is a host with a poor immune system ideal for these creatures, they also thrive on sugar.[2][3] I don't have a normal immune system; I believe that is why I became inundated with them. I believe it should be a common practice for those with chronic diseases to get checked for parasites. According to Dr. Oz, "These hosts rob your body of nutrients." I don't know about you, but I can't afford to lose any more.

---

[2]   Wilson, Lawrence, MD, "Parasites, and How to Eliminate Them Naturally," March 2011, accessed July 12, 2012, http://drlwilson.com/Articles/PARASITES.HTM.

[3]   Dr. Oz Fans, Dr. Oz: Parasites Causing Your Fatigue? Parasite Warning Signs, February 28, 2012, accessed 23 July 2012, http://www.drozfans.com/dr-ozs-advice/dr-oz-parasites-causing-your-fatigue-parasite-warning-signs/.

These are some of the symptoms of parasitic worms:

• Abdominal pain	• Colitis	• Vaginitis	• Muscle spasms
• Hemoptysis	Coughing	• Hair loss or thinning	Insomnia
• Dysuria	Diarrhea	• Joint Pain	• Skin ulcers
• Jaundice	• Digestive disturbance	• Weight loss due to malnutrition	• Rectal prolaspe
• Central nervous system impairment	• Dizziness	• Weakness	• Mental problems
• Chest pain	• Fever	Immuno deficiency	• Lung congestion
• Chills	• Enlargement of various organs	Nausea/ vomit-ing	• Memory loss
• Chronic fatigue	• Headaches	Swelling of facial features	• Night sweats

I have all of those symptoms and then some, which is why I've been unable to exercise with consistency or stand in the kitchen for more than fifteen minutes to fix something nutritious to eat. Please, my autoimmune family, get checked for parasitic worms!

Day 9: Thursday

Concerned about these intestinal infiltrators, I purchase an over-the-counter medication to get rid of the worms and a holistic tonic to get rid of the eggs. I must say, I now know how Sigourney Weaver felt in the movie *Aliens*; what comes out of me could terrorize everyone in that James Cameron movie. Even though I am usually squeamish when it comes to creepy crawlies, the grossness factor of the worms coming out of me isn't an issue because I feel really, really good! My family shares in my excitement of feeling good—but they still won't allow my descriptive ramblings of my poop and infestations.

Day 10: Friday

I feel awesome! Finally! It has been years since I've felt this good. I have no problem standing in the kitchen for long periods of time slicing and dicing fruits and veggies. My dietary habits over the past ten days, coupled with the fact that I disposed of those slimy monsters, make me wonder what other medical issues I would have developed had I not rid my body of the worms. What else does a discombobulated immune system produce? I am too excited right now; I will Google that question later.

After all my efforts to clean out my body, I have enough energy to exercise consistently and am able to follow my dietician's instructions. It is important for me to remember that food is here to sustain me, not to feed an unhealthy addiction of any kind. "Carol," I tell myself, "you can live without the processed junk and the fried foods."

On one occasion, I remember telling my mom, whom I believe is a food addict, about a lunch date I had with a friend of mine. My neighbor had just undergone bariatric surgery; she barely ate what was on her plate. I finally asked her why she ate so meagerly. She explained to me that she was unable to eat large portions because her stomach had been surgically made smaller. The repercussions of overeating after bariatric surgery could be disastrous. I told my mom about this, and she replied, "I would rather die than have any eating restrictions." At first, her comment left me dumfounded. But then I realized my mom's comment probably reflected how most people feel. She was being honest. We want to live life the way we want to live it, but the problem with this philosophy is that most of us don't want to face the consequences of giving into heavy hedonism.

After my ten-day cleanse, I felt wonderful. I reflected on the past, all those years of intermittently feeling ill and what my future would look like. What if I staunchly follow the FDA's daily allowance recommendations as if my life depended on it? What if I drink at least eight glasses of water per day and eat four cups of a combination of fruits and vegetables daily? It is recommended that certain sweets and fats are eaten only sparingly, but is this recommendation for healthy, nondiseased folks? Should I even eat them at all? If I choose to not eat nutritiously, can I then blame my doctor for not doing enough to make me feel better? Is the onus primarily on me? I am afraid these are questions I can't Google. I must look inward. I will pensively search for these answers while eating a hot fudge brownie sundae with caramel and nut toppings. I am kidding (sort of). It is a struggle, but I must remember that feeling good should invariably trump the brief moment of satisfying a craving.

MUST DOs THROUGHOUT THE TEN DAYS

1. Eat fresh vegetables, fruits, raw nuts (with no added sugar or honey), easily digestible fish (e.g., thin slices of smoked salmon, tilapia)
   **If you do not like fish or are concerned about the iodine for those who are hyperthyroid, eat baked chicken but keep the portions small.

2. ABSOLUTELY NO caffeine, sugar of any kind, fruit juices, vegetable juices, alcohol, processed foods, dairy, breads, oats, muffins, or pasta.
3. Take fiber every day.
4. Take calcium and magnesium every day (space it out so you are taking these minerals at least four hours from when you take your thyroid medication.
5. Drink eight to ten glasses of water each day.
6. You may want to halt your exercise regime throughout the cleansing process.

7. Get plenty of rest. You may experience extreme fatigue throughout this process. That's okay, as those toxins are working their way out of you.
8. Take hot baths.
9. Balance your fruit, vegetable, and protein intake. In other words, don't eat just apples or peas all day because those are the only cleanse-approved foods you like. Eat a balanced blend throughout the day.

• Remember: Day one or day two (depending on the person) is very difficult. Pray you get through it, and keep at it. It will be worth it in the end.

If you want to try this ten-day cleanse, I want to support you! E-mail me at CrazyThyroidLady@gmail.com any time for questions, comments, venting, or support.

After the cleanse, I felt well enough to move forward with my dietician's meal plan. I had the energy to consistently exercise, and I had also incorporated drinking noni juice (I do not endorse or sell any particular noni juice product). I am proud to say that these efforts have allowed me to lose a significant amount of weight. And let me tell you, after radioactive iodine therapy, losing weight (without cleansing) was nearly impossible.

The noni juice was a great MacGraver enhancement. According to Neil Solomon, MD, PhD, a Johns Hopkins-trained physician and *New York Times* best-selling author of *The Noni Solution,* there are three reasons why noni juice helps with weight loss:

1. It is rich in antioxidants.
2. It gives you more energy to move and burn off calories.
3. The noni fruit contains a substance called xeronine. After studying the benefits of noni for more than a decade, Dr. Solomon explains in his book how xeronine works to enhance sick cells in the body. For more information about

noni juice and its weight-loss and medicinal properties, check out these sources:

- http://www.nonijuicecentral.com/noni_research.pdf
- *The Noni Solution* by Neil Solomon MD, PhD
- http://www.nothingbutnoni.com/nonifaqs.aspx
- *76 Ways to Use Noni Fruit Juice* by Isa Navarre

Chapter 5

Family and Friends

There's always that one episode in every television series in which a family conflict is the central theme. And even though MacGyver could singlehandedly take out the bad guys with a ballpoint pen and a paper clip, he was not immune to the inescapable family drama. In episode ten of season one, MacGyver reunites with his long-lost grandfather, who had reared him and with whom MacGyver had not spoken in many years. In the beginning of the episode, it becomes apparent that a deep-rooted disagreement had divided these two men. But by the end, both grandfather and son have to come together to get out of one of MacGyver's predicaments. The pair realized they need to accept each other and work harmoniously for the greater good.

My original plan for this book did not include a chapter about friends and family. It is not that they aren't important to me; it's just that I've always been reluctant to bring others on board my burden bus. Subsequent to my diagnosis, my rigid conviction epitomizes the ignorance I had about thyroid disease. Even now, I still struggle with the fact that those close to me *must* share in this inconsistent, tumultuous battle in life and on these pages. Their inclusion is practical, whether I like it or not.

Unfortunately, making the decision to continually keep all those aggravating symptoms hidden from those who are nearest and dearest can bring about negative reactions aimed at the sufferer. I myself have been the recipient of disdain, criticism, scorn, and on occasion, downright repulsion for acting like a "lazy slob." They don't understand what not feeling well means, that if someone were to put a gun to my head, I still would not be motivated enough to get up and do the dishes. After all, to our friends and family, we thyroid sufferers look fine for the most part. The term "invisible illness" fits, doesn't it? So, in some cases, even if you do tell friends or family members how you really feel, your "at death's door" descriptions may go in one ear and out the other. But hey, you can say you tried.

Society has been conditioned to believe that symptoms such as chronic pain, fatigue, and brain fog are only reserved for the elderly, or those who have cancer, suffer from COPD, or have severe musculoskeletal diseases. In fact, I remember one occasion, while I was working at The Pit, when a group of employees (comprised primarily of managers) was in the boardroom preparing for a meeting. I had been asked to take down the meeting's minutes. The meeting took place shortly after my Graves' disease diagnosis but *before* the RAI treatment. Needless to say, I was in bad shape. Looking back, I don't know how I was functional enough to drive into work and sit upright for an entire workday. No doubt, I had special angels working around the clock to keep me from falling into a manhole or wandering around an airport hundreds of miles away in another state.

There we were, sitting around the boardroom table and awaiting the arrival of the director of behavioral health. The typical informal chitchatting ensued in an effort to avoid awkward silence gaps. One manager asked the administrator how one of the other directors was doing. She had been gone on a leave of absence after undergoing chemotherapy for breast cancer. The administrator hesitantly looked around the room and, after realizing that we were all caring coworkers, decided it would be okay to give a health status report.

"She is doing fine, her energy is coming back, but her chief complaint is brain fog," she said.

"Oh, my goodness. I definitely can relate to that," I added with automated excitement.

Everyone in the room knew of my disease diagnosis. Not only had I missed a lot of work, but my voice had been hoarse too, like a mix between Carol Channing and Rachel Ray. I had become so rail thin that my clothes were falling off me, and my hand tremors were Parkinson's-like. My condition did not stop any of them from shooting nasty, piercing eyeball-daggers my way. *How dare you compare yourself to someone with cancer?* I was in no way trying to be insensitive to my coworker's cancer plight; it was just that at that moment I could relate to the immense case of brain fog that thyroid disorders bring. Also, my Graves' disease had been so bad that, if had I gone without treatment much longer, I might not have made it. But, again, trying to compare the afflictions of both diseases is an exercise in futility. The truth is, no one can truly know what another person is going through.

Fortunately, though, not having a fully functional brain can sometimes be a good thing; the disdain that those women had for me at that moment did not register until later on that evening. By then I was too sick and tired to ruminate over it. Had I comprehended their hateful glares while in the moment, I probably would have burst into hysterical tears. The waterworks could flow fast and furious before my radioactive treatment, but that incident was my first taste of being the recipient of judgment by others who believe that a person can't suffer, unless they have a common, well-known disease.

I was too brain fogged to tell my coworkers about one particular incident that occurred at the grocery store. I couldn't find my car in the parking lot. Doesn't sound that uncommon, does it? Well, it was. Not only could I not find where I had parked, I couldn't remember what kind of car I drove. Flashes of all the cars, I had ever driven in my life, including my first car (which I had gotten when I was seventeen years old) ran through my mind. I just couldn't remember which one had taken me to the store that day. What a frightening moment. Unfortunately, I did not think to give this account to my critical colleagues, but fast-on-your-feet thinking is not common for those with thyroid dysfunction. It's probably just as well; they might not have believed that a thirtysomething could have had this experience.

—

I felt compelled to write this chapter because my sister and mother (with whom I am very close) and I got into an argument one day. An argument among the three of us is a rarity. I can count on one hand the serious disagreements we have had. The main reason we rarely clash is because we are very open and honest with our feelings. Most issues don't get swept under the rug—except of course the daily difficulties I face living with an autoimmune thyroid disease and my family's seeming lack of concern. I became extremely hurt after one incident, and my deep pain made me realize I had harbored some resentment that I had to let it out.

It all started one Friday. (Pretend like this is a movie dream sequence; I so love those.) Working thyroidians do cherish their Fridays, probably more than the average person does. Anyway, neither my sister nor my mother works outside of the home. My sister is a stay-at-home mom, and my mother is retired. I work forty to forty-five hours a week, so not only am I an employee, I'm also a wife, mother, cook, chauffer, family manager—and at the same time, I'm trying to figure out how to control a cryptic disease. Cooking for an hour or so after work means there is little time left for myself and for my family before I go to bed and then wake up to do it all over again. Fridays are usually my noncooking days. I typically arrive home from work and pass out like a drunken sailor onto anything cushy.

My sister and mom have a habit of calling me everyday, which is fine; it's been going on all my life. After the death of my father, however, they began calling me multiple times a day (probably another reason I grabbed junk food). And the calls were insane! I am talking restraining-order insane. I would take these calls (while at work) and try to act pleasant just to keep the peace because I knew both were having a hard time. But all the while, a large vein in my forehead would pulsate. For a thyroid-disease sufferer, getting disrupted while in the midst of concentrated work efforts is like a worm being taken many feet away from its little wormhole; it could take hours, perhaps days, to get back to the starting position.

My boss and I were working closely together one Friday to prepare for an approaching audit; this forced me to ignore my mom and sister's phone calls all day. The stress of this upcoming audit gave my boss a bad cold. Since my immune system was not cooperating anymore, I began to feel puny toward the end of the day; I was catching her cold. If someone is sick and within a few feet of me, chances are, I'll catch it, especially if I am not actively using all my MacGraver's tricks. I did not take my mom and sister's calls all weekend because I was in bed convalescing; this was imperative so that I could make it back to work on Monday. When I called them both on Monday to check in, each gave me chilly *Mean Girl* attitudes. I thought, *Are we in high school?*

One thing about having a chronic disease, I've found, is that the bull caca you once tolerated, becomes intolerable. I had to let them know that they must cease and desist with the nonstop calling. During working hours, I demanded that they text or e-mail me if they wanted to ask questions like, "What are you having for dinner tonight?" or "What is the name of that lotion you used that made your hands so soft?" These types of telephone inquiries were not acceptable anymore. I was firm and blunt, yet calm, with my instructions. This new rule meant I wouldn't have to hurt anyone's feelings if I was unable to answer phone calls because I was busy or convalescing.

MacGraver's Tip

If it is easier to write letters to let your friends or family members know how much stress they are unnecessarily putting on you, then by all means, get your point across that way no matter how cheesy it seems. What matters is letting your feelings be known. It is not selfishness. It is

self-preservation, and your family must understand this.
Stand your ground. They will come around.

━

I have found that in order for me to truly live with this disease
alongside my friends and family, I am going to have to evolve from
one crazy to another, what I call "comfortably crazy." I understand
there are those who are very sensitive to the word *crazy* because of
all the negative emotions it evokes. Plus, you were probably called
crazy or treated like you were by several health-care professionals
while you were seeking your thyroid disorder diagnosis.

I'll admit to jumping out of my skin when someone entered
the room, crying during mundane conversations with people,
maintaining a daily zombie-like disposition; these actions all
occurred pretreatment. I probably would not have been crowned
Ms. Sanity of the Year, but I am not ashamed of this. I was sick, and
those were my symptoms. It saddens me that other thyroid-disease
sufferers don't want to speak out about the cognitive symptoms that
accompany their illnesses. It also saddens me that friends and family
will call thyroid-malfunctioning people crazy, as if this is okay to say.
Would you call someone with a bad leg a "lame cripple" to his face?
They don't realize how hurtful it can be to point out an imperfection
due to an incurable disease or defect. But their mocking hurts. So,
with a lot of hard work and MacGraver tricks, I've turned my crazy
into something positive, the kind of crazy that will help me to deal
with the folks who can hurt you the most.

What does my new *crazy* look like?

C

C stands for **comfort**. Get comfortable with your disease. I know
this must sound strange, like I am telling you to acquiesce to the

illness. You *should* fight to feel better, but don't fight with the disease. Educate yourself. *What is this disease doing to my body from the ankle to my zygomatic bone?* Don't be in denial. Accept the hand that is dealt, and work toward living comfortably.

C also stands for **common**. Find others who are in your shoes. I know how difficult it is to be surrounded by friends and family who have no idea what it is like to suffer from this disease. MacGraver mentioned support groups in a previous chapter, and I must reiterate how important it is to share your feelings with similar individuals who can give understanding and support.

Lastly, *C* stands for **conserving**. This is very important because getting stressed out and angry with your friends and family takes a lot of energy. It's best to let them know how you feel calmly, but sternly, and then move on. Conserving energy is key when you have a thyroid disease because fatigue is a primary symptom. If I know ahead of time a family outing is coming up on a weekend. I try to cut back on other activities throughout the week, so that I can be well rested for any future events.

R

R stands for **remove**. Remove anything that sucks the life right out of you. Remember the old movie *The Blob*? That black-and-white movie terrified me as a child. Imagine some sort of large Jell-O mold is consuming you and there is nothing you can do about it . . . Chilling! Thinking about it still gives me goose bumps. Imagine the negative, disparaging, and emotionally draining people as that Jell-O mold, suffocating the life right out of you. Chronic disease sufferers need to keep their distance from these folks. I know this may be difficult, but if your health has completely deteriorated, you are no good to anyone, including the ones who *don't* suck.

That topic segues to my next *R*, **revive.** Revive those relationships with folks who do make you feel good, those who lift you up and make you feel good about yourself. *R* also stands for **resolute**. Be firm with those around you. If you don't feel well and are unable to do something on a certain day, let your loved ones know. If it seems they aren't taking no for an answer, let them know exactly what is going on with your body. It is better to do this than to lie and then not show up. Again, less drama and stress. **Reveal** who you are, don't put on airs. Lastly, *R* stands for **restoring**. I think about restoring a piece of art, a car, or furniture. There is a lot of mending, painting, gluing, and fixing going on. This is what we are doing to ourselves, and this is what this book is about. Coming up with ways to get back to, close to, or better than where you were before.

Conserving and Restoring

Adding

Z

Z stands for **zeal** or **zest**. Conserving and restoring yourself will hopefully add more energy and sharpness. If I do these things, I can hang with my friends and family members for a few hours more than if I had been running around hectically prior to the outing.

IN

YOU

Bottom line, this is *your* body and *your* disease. Those close to you share in this with you, but at the end of the day only you know what it feels like! Most of the time, I would not wish my disease on my worst enemy, but to be honest, there are other days when I say to myself, "I really wish [insert name here] could feel what I go through for just one hour." Then, I come to my senses and realize God allowed me to go through this because He knew I could handle it.

You can ask my family and friends if I ascribe to the above philosophy, and they will surely say *yes*. I would recommend that all of my thyroid brothers and sisters *go crazy*!

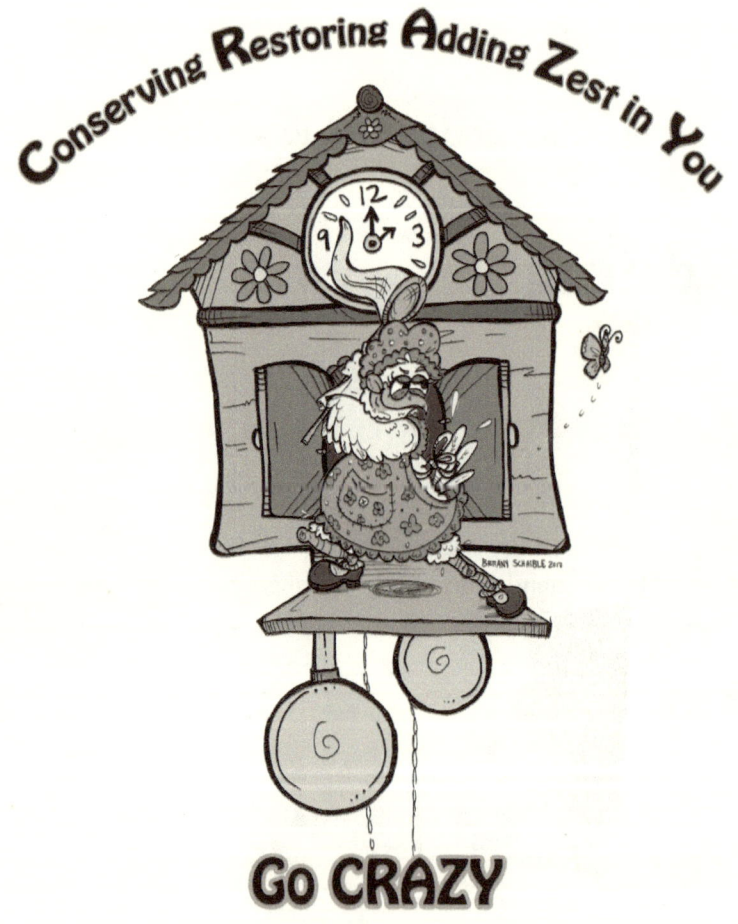

**A brief intermission to share a tip from a MacGraver friend who also has Graves' disease, Elizabeth.

THERAPY! I lost my father at the same time I was diagnosed and had RAI; and without seeking out a therapist, I would have plunged into a downward spiral. Seriously owe my life to her!

I also went to many different endos until I found one that I honestly believed knew what he was talking about and was concerned with ME and not just numbers. He was the one that suggested me trying selenium and making me a little hyper, which has improved my quality of life dramatically.

After three years, I don't really suffer from any side effects at all. I feel normal and back to my pre-GD diagnosis, and I'm HAPPY.

Chapter 5

The Next Generation

I've asked the two most important people in my life and the poor souls who are "lucky" enough to get an up close and personal view of my disease, to give their insights on what it is like to live with a thyroid-disease sufferer:

My Husband

I have known Carol for over twenty years, and we have been married nineteen-plus at the time of this writing. In the course of her book she might not have expanded on some things about herself that I would like you to know. Carol is not eager to show her profile picture on her blogs and social networking sites because she wants to represent herself as "every woman" with this disease. However, Carol is very beautiful (both inside and out). She has a sort of "ageless" face that will treat her well as she grows into her elderly years; that same face, however, also represented her well during her younger years as a model. It is a wonder that we have remained married, because like most couples, we've had our fair share of struggles, almost resulting in a divorce. Admittedly, most of our marital problems have stemmed from problems I have created and not because of her disease. One thing I know for certain is that the sole reason she wrote this book was to help *you*, the chronic disease sufferer.

Throughout most of her disease, and especially in the beginning stages, I did not give her the attention she deserved. Unfortunately for her (and my son), I was also "suffering" but in a different sort of way. Battling a progressively worse painkiller addiction for the better part of six years, in my own selfish way, had me focused mainly on one thing: me. Or should I say, the need for my next high.

My disease would not allow me to care much about anything except figuring out how I was going to get my next fix. Not that I was a terrible person, because I don't think I was. I always treasured my wife and son; it's just that I could not put any of their needs above mine.

Now that I am sober, I look back on that time period with a tremendous amount of guilt and regret. I have always been, by all accounts, a laid-back guy on the outside but deeply complex—or maybe even a perplexed person—on the inside. Through the years, I have never inflicted any physical harm to my family, but because I was locked inside myself, I know that I have caused them much undo mental pain. By placing myself above them, I have spent way too much of our money on drugs and, to some extent, gambling. For the most part, however, to the average onlooker, I would not come across as a lowlife degenerate.

I always managed to get by with what could be viewed as "functional" addict behavior. Between our two incomes, we have lived most of our marriage in the middle to upper-middle income bracket. Most of our money was spent faster than we could make it, and it seems like usually we were in a good deal of debt. This was especially true during the last four or five years when my income went down but my insatiable appetite for drugs got out of hand.

Because of my own deplorable behavior, I could hardly notice when Carol was in the beginning stages of her sickness. Initially, I did notice that she would spend countless hours of her free time in bed just resting or mostly sleeping. She would always complain that there was something wrong with her that could not be diagnosed.

In my mind, I was pretty much under the assumption that she was a hypochondriac.

Early in our marriage, she had her share of sicknesses and ailments, such as chronic sinusitis, heart problems, and bladder infections, to name a few. I thought her issues were signs of hypochondria. However, some—if not most—of these things *did* lead to treatment and/or surgeries, so I do know that they were not made up in her head.

As for the Graves' disease, it is just now in the last year or so that I have come to accept and respect what she has gone through. Like I said, at the onset of her disease, she would mostly lie in bed complaining about something that was wrong that no doctor could fix. At times, in addition to the oversleeping, she would be very hyper and could not sit still or sleep much. Also, I do recall with clarity her unwillingness to give up on finding what was causing her so many problems. I know she has outlined these episodes in this book. Hypo versus hyper is something I have learned about from her disease over the last year, and I know it is not make-believe.

I have seen the great dedication she has devoted over the past several years to being well, documenting all of her trials and tribulations, all in an effort to bring to you some helpful hints, if not solutions, to what you are going through. She did not write this book to gain any sort of fortune or fame. It was borne out of her dealing with this disease and all the frustration of doctors not knowing how to treat it.

I have learned a lot about autoimmune disease during her fight. I know everything she has put into this book was designed to help you. I wish I had been more sympathetic toward her plight in the beginning, but now I find myself fully on board and in support of everything she is trying to do to bring about solutions and awareness for this disease. She is a beautiful woman in so many ways, and I am very blessed to have her love, and I know for sure that she loves you too!

My Son

My mom asked me to write about how I feel about the disease she has. I really don't want to do this, because my favorite TV show is on right now and this is like schoolwork. But I told her I would write something, so I did.

Chapter 6

Cautionary Tales, Take Care of You

What happens when you ignore your doctor's advice or, more important, what your body is telling you?

The following are three cautionary tales of thyroid sufferers who succumbed to the dangers of thyroid disease when it was not properly treated. That little butterfly gland can do so much harm, as you will see.

Yang Bing, 51

Yang Bing was diagnosed with Graves' disease and began taking a drug to inhibit the thyroid hormone from being overproduced in his body. After more than five years, he decided to stop taking the prescribed medication without consulting with his physician.

Shortly after he stopped, his legs and hands began to swell. Not only did they swell, but he also developed a hard, shell-like layer of skin, creating sort of a *Michelin-man* type ring surrounding his entire body. Pictures of part of Mr. Bing's body can be found on the internet.

Gail Devers, 46

Gail Devers is a three-time medalist Olympic track runner in 1992 and 1996. She dazzled all who watched her glide around the track, and she was touted as one of the fastest female runners in the world. Ms. Devers made a name for herself not just because of her speed but also because of her long *Edward Scissorhands*-like nails, which became her signature. Gail was diagnosed in 1990 with Graves' disease. She quickly learned that it does not matter how muscular, strong, and fast you are, diseases can sometimes take the upper hand.

Prior to Gail's diagnosis she had been under a lot of stress. She was planning a marriage, dealing with a demanding coach, and also trying to stay in Olympic shape. It sounds like she had a lot of stress weight on her shoulders. According to the Lifetime network made-for-TV movie about her life, *Run for the Dream,* a medication prescribed by her doctor to help control some of her Graves' symptoms, was on the list of substances banned by the Olympic committee. Keeping it a secret, Gail decided to not take the much-needed medication. This decision turned out to be near-fatal for her.

After deciding to forgo the medication, Gail began to notice her lightning speed on the track disappearing. She became irritable, and her marriage started to crumble. She began to isolate herself because she did not want anyone to see the visible deterioration of this once athletically built woman. She developed severe swelling in her legs and feet to the point that doctors thought they would have to amputate Gail's legs. Such irony that the two things that had made Gail a rising star were the very things that were almost taken away due to her desire to run at all costs.

Thankfully, Gail's legs were saved, and her health and fitness were restored to Olympic-level status again. She went on to receive more gold medals after this major setback. Her celebrity prominence allowed Gail to have a platform. On January 26, 2000, Gail testified before Congress imploring for better education within the medical and scientific community as to the horror and dangers of thyroid diseases that are left untreated or are mismanaged.

Gail's health scare is definitely a cautionary tale, but also ultimately a story she turned into a triumph. She is truly one of my heroes.

Judy Kirby, 43

One Saturday afternoon, on March 25, 2000, Judy Kirby drove up an access road, heading the wrong way on a busy highway. As a result, she killed seven people, including four of her own children. Her defense attorneys believed multiple causes contributed to this tragic accident, among them that she had just given birth to her eighth child five months earlier and had exhibited postpartum depression symptoms. Her family said her demeanor had completely changed and she had become unrecognizable after the birth of her baby girl. The other contributing factor, according to her lawyers, was a mismanaged thyroid disorder.

Weeks before this freeway tragedy, Judy was taken by ambulance to the hospital because she complained of breathing problems. Following a quick assessment, she was immediately taken to the behavioral health unit where she had been given an initial diagnosis of postpartum psychosis. Risperdal, a psychotic drug, was administered upon her arrival. Her TSH (thyroid stimulating hormone) levels were very low, indicating hyperthyroidism. The on-call psychiatrist was just eight months out of residency and, according to Judy's defense, did not do a thorough job to see if perhaps her psychotic displays were thyroid related and not due to postpartum depression. The psychiatrist did not think Judy's symptoms were related to her thyroid even though the doctor admitted that her TSH and T3 levels were very low. She did not conduct further sensitive thyroid function tests because she said "physically" Judy did not show signs of a thyroid dysfunction during her two-day stay at the hospital. The psychiatrist gave Judy Zoloft for her depression and lowered her Synthroid dosage. However, Judy's psychosis made her very paranoid, and due to her distrust of the doctor, she did not take the new Synthroid dosage after leaving the hospital. Judy continued taking the other higher dosage of Synthroid prescribed previously by her primary doctor.

Judy's friends and family testified at trial that her psychotic symptoms continued shortly after the hospital stay weeks prior to the fatal collision. I regularly speak to Judy, who is now behind bars, but she does not remember the day of the accident, which is understandable because of the state she was in at the time and the fact that she suffered a brain injury, resulting in a coma after the accident. Judy is currently serving a 215-year sentence because the prosecution said that someone would only drive the wrong way for 1.7 miles if she were trying to kill herself.

This is a tragic story and one of the main reasons I became such a staunch thyroid advocate. This could have been me. At my sickest, prior to proper treatment, I could have easily driven the wrong way on a busy highway. Psychosis can definitely make a person thoroughly confused or out of touch with reality. It is imperative that all health-care providers understand and realize the devastating effects that can occur if thyroid dysfunction of any kind is left unmanaged or is not completely tested to find out the exact reason for the malfunction. I will detail Judy Kirby's life in my second book, *Sentenced for Sickness, 215 Years: The Judy Kirby Story.*

Again, I implore you, don't take your thyroid disorder lightly. As you can see from the stories above, thyroid disease needs to be managed properly and vigilantly. Take care of you!

**The story will continue right after this message from my MacGraver friend, Tyrone, who has polymyositis.

In late April of 2010 I began to have several symptoms that led to me being diagnosed with polymyositis in June of 2010. Polymyositis is a type of myositis. Myositis is a general term for inflammation of the muscles. Many such conditions are considered likely to be caused by autoimmune conditions. Because of this, I have had to develop many ways of coping with this disease. First of all, I now take thirteen to fifteen different medications, which include insulin, on a daily basis. I also take a Methotrexate (chemotherapy) injection once a week.

I also no longer work due to the daily fatigue and pain I endure daily. So I have been trying to garden on a daily basis just to keep some kind of activity in place. And the times that I have not been able to garden, I've been exercising in the pool and gym. Aqua therapy really helped me mentally and physically when I was unable to have any movement whatsoever. I've also tried to do as much housework as possible to help out my wife while she is working. But I must take multiple breaks whenever I do this housework. Leaning on God and my friends and family has given me peace while learning to cope with polymyositis.

People don't realize how much pets can help a person cope with disease and sickness. My cats have been a tremendous help to me. And one other thing that has helped me cope with polymyositis is social media. I am a member of several myositis and polymyositis Facebook pages and have even developed several friendships from social media. I even have a mentor who has had polymyositis for seven years and helped me work through many of the hurdles that come with polymyositis.

Chapter 7

The Twelve Steps
for the Thyroid Sufferer

In the midst of my working at The Pit and trying to manage this wretched disease, my husband was in a battle of his own: the challenging disease of addiction. The severity of his addiction had grown in such a way that I knew I had to do something or I would lose him. With much agonizing deliberation and prayer, I made a decision to expose what he had been trying to hide. I staged an intervention with his family. This confrontation came on the heels of my father's death, which made the situation even more painful. Losing my father and the possibility of losing my husband had me contemplating whether I would be strong enough to make it through.

In order to give my husband the help he needed while still taking care of myself, I knew I needed to strengthen my mind, my body, and also my spirituality. The situation had to be completely turned over to God. This meant no worries, no strife, and no fear—just complete unadulterated faith. Faith that He would work it out for my good. Oh, how much freedom is felt when you give Him your burdens! This was *weight* that only my heavenly Father could carry; I had to hand it over.

After the intervention, my husband agreed to check himself into an in-patient rehabilitation facility for a week of treatment. After his release, he then participated in intensive outpatient therapy three nights a week for six weeks. As a family unit, my son and I accompanied him to a meeting one night a week throughout those six weeks. I praise God my husband embraced the weeklong rehabilitation stay, as well as the meetings, sponsors, literature, and books. There is definitely a gradual therapeutic process to staying clean and sober, and a big part of an addict's successful journey is contingent upon whether or not they follow this twelve-step program.

The core foundation of the twelve steps is the belief in a higher power. The higher power (God) is who addicts lean on for strength and guidance as they work through their disease.

I was happy to support my husband's sobriety, and while I was attending a Narcotics Anonymous meeting, it dawned on me that the twelve-step program that has been used to help those with additive diseases for many decades was something I could apply to my disease battle. Hence, these twelve steps for the thyroid sufferer were inspired by those principles:

1. **We admit we have some power over our illness and that we *can* be involved in the management of the disease.**

For the addict, the first step is admitting that you are powerless over your addiction. In the thyroid sufferer's first step, we must admit that we *do have* some power in our healing. Even though I know most of you feel as if you are powerless when dealing with your health-care professional, I am beseeching you now to take control of your health. You must sternly tell your primary health-care professional (and others) that you deserve to feel better than you do.

I have a hard time accepting the fact that I can no longer eat White Castle hamburgers at three in the morning or a bag of Lifesavers gummies in minutes without any consequences (well, without any consequences that were known to me, before my diagnosis). Maybe it wasn't a good idea to start those bad habits in the first place. There are so many reasons why I ate imprudently. I don't want to place the blame on anyone except myself, but media reports advising that it is okay to eat junk food "occasionally" weren't the best directive for me. "Occasionally" is a relative term isn't it? My *occasionally* is once or twice a week, and what if this occasional eating of food with little or no nutritional value was one of the contributors to my autoimmune disease? What would happen if we *occasionally* put water in our gas tanks?

We must take control of our health by placing great emphasis on what we *should* consume, as well as finding out if we have any food sensitivities and avoiding these things. There are tests for this. Journal in a food diary to see what makes you sick and what gives you energy. What I can eat might not be the same things you can eat. Take the time to prepare fresh fruits and veggies on a daily basis. You can do it!

Also you should regularly keep track of how you feel. Research and find out what vitamin and mineral supplements you may need to add to your diet. Thyroid-disease sufferers should seek out supplements that chiefly aid heart health, metabolism, bones, and brain function.

I remember when I first read the Bible verse below and how much it impacted me. I am housing something within me that is very important. It was given to me by God; therefore I must take care of myself.

> *1 Corinthians 6:19-20* "Don't you realize that your body is the temple of the Holy Spirit, who lives in you and was given to you by God? You do not belong to yourself, for God bought you with a high price. So you must honor God with your body."

2. Believe that a Power greater than ourselves can restore us to sanity.

There are so many neurological issues associated with thyroid disease: anxiety, depression, brain fog, irritability . . . the list goes on and on. What is misunderstood by most people (including most doctors) is that these symptoms are organic and typically not a result of our stressful environments. So in other words, a thyroid sufferer could be in the middle of Shangri-la with not a care in the world and still feel anxious, depressed, and irritable. Organic just means that these symptoms are brought on by a neurochemical, neuroendocrinologic, structural, or other *physical* impairment. I believe God ordains doctors and medicine to help us with our well-being. If neurological medication is needed for you to control these symptoms, by all means take it; but you and I both know medication isn't enough sometimes. This is why continuous efforts to stay close to your Higher Power are important to gain spiritual strength.

In the beginning states of their treatment, many drug addicts are prescribed medication to help fight withdrawal, but they are still plugged into the twelve-step principles for spiritual strength.

> **2 Corinthians 12:9** "My grace is sufficient for you, for my *power* is made perfect in weakness."

3. Make a decision to turn our will and our lives over to the *care* of God as we understand Him.

This is the exact verbiage for step number three. I did not alter a word because it is so fitting. God is the ultimate caregiver, the Great Physician, so collaborate with Him first with regard to your care. I am not a religious zealot who believes in no medications, no doctors, and no hospitals. Some believe this is the only way to show your faith in God. Again, I believe God has a hand in the creation of those who are here to make us well. What I glean from the third step is that God wants us to seek him first when it comes to our health and wellness. In other words, pray before you seek out a health-care professional. Pray for discernment for yourself, pray for wisdom for the one treating you, and most important, pray for strength. Life is hard. Life with an illness is even harder, but having the Primary primary care physician at your disposal means all things are possible, including having a better disposition about your affliction. Include Him in your treatment plan.

> **1 Peter 5:7** "Cast all your anxiety on him because he cares for you."

4.   Make a searching and fearless inventory of ourselves.

Throughout my disease journey, I have met so many amazing, wonderful people who refuse to talk about their disease publically. Their reasoning: "I don't want this disease to define who I am." I don't understand this way of thinking. How can talking about something you are afflicted with define who you are? You are who you are, period. You have the illness whether you want to talk about it or not. If you do, however, communicate with others about it, then perhaps you can offer advice, recommend a doctor, or just offer a shoulder to cry on. It is not about complaining or whining about your disease; it's about empowering yourself and others with support and information. Whatever is illuminated within our persona and not suppressed, I believe is an area in which we are asking God to help us. The truth can set you free.

> **John 8:32** "Then you will know the truth, and the truth will set you free."

5.   Admit to ourselves and others our capabilities.

You are a strong person to be surviving thyroid disease. It is not easy. When one symptom seems to dissipate, another may rear its ugly head. Even though you exude a lot of courage in dealing with this difficult disease, don't forget to take care of yourself and understand your limitations. We live in an age in which multitasking and high-octane workloads are applauded. I don't think God intended for us to keep up at the busy pace that some of us have welcomed into our lives. Sickness can sometimes be your body's way of telling you to slow down.

Take a look at this portion of the Twenty-Third Psalm:

[1] The LORD is my shepherd, I shall not be in want.
[2] He *makes me lie down* in green pastures,
    he leads me beside quiet waters,

³ he restores my soul.
   He guides me in paths of righteousness
   for his name's sake.
⁴ Even though I walk
   through the valley of the shadow of death,
   I will fear no evil,
   for you are with me;
   your rod and your staff,
   they comfort me.

Let the Lord lead you throughout life's journey. He is your shepherd; he knows when you need to lie down in green pastures and when He must lead you beside quiet waters. He can restore you to peace that surpasses all understanding if you call on Him.

6. We're entirely ready to accept this season that God has put us in.

As an autoimmune-disease sufferer, I never know what the day will bring. Will I roll a lucky number seven or throw snake eyes and crap out? Not knowing how your body will behave from day to day is frustrating to say the least. It's not an easy way to live, and in my darkest moments I would often ask myself, *Why me?* Then quickly I would recall lectures I had given to my son when he was younger. After he had faced a difficult day and asked that same question, I would say, "Why *not* you?" Fortunately or unfortunately (it depends on how you want to view it), none of us is immune to life's challenges. God has brought you to this chapter in your life for a reason, but despite what you may think sometimes, He will not give you more than you can handle.

> **2 Corinthians 4:16-18** "Therefore we do not lose heart. Though outwardly we are wasting away, yet inwardly we are being renewed day by day. ¹⁷ For our light and momentary troubles are achieving for us an eternal glory that far outweighs them all. ¹⁸ So we fix our eyes not on

what is seen, but on what is unseen, since what is seen is temporary, but what is unseen is eternal."

7. Ask God to give us strength daily

Since God is unseen it is hard, even for the strongest of Christians, to remember to call on him for strength every day. He can quiet your mind and remind you to pull out those MacGraver's tricks if needed, stay calm and level headed, eat nutritionally . . . The list goes on and on. Whatever you need, He is there to deliver if you are willing and receptive.

> **Isaiah 40:31** "But those who hope in the Lord will renew their strength. They will soar on the wings like eagles; they will run and not grow weary, they will walk and not be faint."

> **Philippians 4:13** "I can do everything through him who gives me strength."

> **Isaiah 40:29** "He gives strength to the weary and increases the power of the weak."

> **Matthew 7:7** "Ask and it will be given to you; seek and you will find; knock and the door will be opened to you."

8. Make a list of those who were unsympathetic to your illness and forgive them, with the help of God.

Forgiveness is powerful. It will also release some of your stress weight. Unnecessary and undue stress has no place in a life of someone who is chronically ill.

> **Proverbs 17:9** "He who covers and forgives an offense seeks love, but he who repeats or harps on a matter separates even close friends."

9.   Make close connections with positive and uplifting influencers.

I don't know about you, but I seem to feel better when I make a conscience effort to be a positive force in someone else's life. Consequently, I want those types of people in my life. It's a win-win for both parties. Unfortunately we cannot completely avoid emotional vampires in our lives, but we can keep them at a distance. Establishing close connections means being careful with the information you are willing to dole out to those who get great pleasure in using what you say against you. It is a game for them. Don't play.

> **Philippians 4:8** "Finally, brothers, whatever is true, whatever is noble, whatever is right, whatever is pure, whatever is lovely, whatever is admirable—if anything is excellent or praiseworthy—think about such things."

10. Take inventory of your shortcomings. Don't take your illness out on someone else.

Irritability and thyroid disease go hand in hand. This is *my* main shortcoming. I have flown off the handle on more than one occasion, and then after my tantrum was over, I've asked myself, "Was that really necessary?" Usually I would ask this question weeks later because in the midst of my irritable state, my psyche was such that I wasn't entirely cognizant of my irritability. More often than not, I look back on my temper tantrums weeks later, embarrassed that I behaved that way. I despise this symptom of my illness. You never know what someone else is going through, so I absolutely don't want to put stress weight on them.

Legitimate anger is not a sin (James 1:19: "My dear brothers and sisters, take note of this: Everyone should be quick to listen, slow to speak and slow to become angry"). Being slow to anger or thinking prior to anger is a virtuous act. But not every action done or said out of anger is legitimate. Take a step back and think before you do or say something you might regret. I know this is easier said than done, but if this is your shortcoming, ask God to help you in this area. If your intention is to work on all your shortcomings with God's help, and not take things out on others, you will garner positive results, *every time*. Remember we are all going through something. Don't believe your struggles trump what is going on with others. Love one another, shortcomings and all.

> **Luke 6:36-38** "Be merciful, just as your Father is merciful. ³⁷ "Do not judge, and you will not be judged. Do not condemn, and you will not be condemned. Forgive, and you will be forgiven. ³⁸ Give, and it will be given to you. A good measure, pressed down, shaken together and running over, will be poured into your lap. For with the measure you use, it will be measured to you."

11. Make time for prayer and meditation.

During the heart of my illness, I honestly could not have made it through those difficult times without prayer and meditation. Thyroid disorder is a neurological disorder, among other things. It has affected me more mentally than physically. With my extreme anxiety, depression, hallucinations, and brain fog, I have had to plug into God daily to lead me out of the shadow of death. Before treatment, this was uncharted territory for me, but the Lord was my seeing-eye dog so to speak, directing me though the uncertainty I felt while I was deeply, mentally sick. Prayer and meditation are very important; they are conversing with, listening to, and acknowledging your Father in heaven.

> **Thessalonians 5:17** "Pray without ceasing."

> **Psalm 19:13-14** "Keep your servant also from willful sins; may they not rule over me. Then will I be blameless, innocent of great transgression. May the words of my mouth and the meditation of my heart be pleasing in your sight, O LORD, my Rock and my Redeemer."

Psalm 39:3-4 "My heart grew hot within me, and as I meditated, the fire burned; then I spoke with my tongue: 'Show me, O LORD, my life's end and the number of my days; let me know how fleeting is my life.'"

12. Help other thyroid suffers get through their illness.

One of God's greatest commandments is to love Him. If we do this with all of our heart, than loving others (His children) will come easily. One way to love others is by helping other thyroid sufferers who may have difficulties getting through? I love all of you and hope and pray this book can aid you in some way. May God bless you and keep you strong.

Philippians 2:4 Let each of you look not only to his own interests, but also to the interests of others.

Chapter 8

Crazy Thyroid Lady's Quick Guide and Other Tips

MacGraver's Quick Guide

Brain Function

1. Drink plenty of water.
2. Drink matcha (green tea powder).
   See "What are the Benefits of Match Green Tea Powder,"
   http://www.livestrong.com/article/282502-what-are-the-
   benefits-of-matcha-green-tea-powder/

3. Get adequate amounts of sleep each night.
4. Make sure your iron levels are normal.
5. Exercise your brain with puzzles, games, and reading.

Eat Nutritionally without Breaking the Bank

1. Get quarter cups or one half cups of *each* vegetable you want at the grocery story deli, if available, instead of buying in bulk.
2. Seek out local farmers markets or produce stands.

3. If you have to purchase bigger quantities, share the cost with neighbors.
4. Grow your own vegetables and fruits.
5. Save produce longer by vacuum sealing it.

Stress

1. Don't forget the four Ps: position, perspective, pressure, and pain.
2. Find positive support groups during difficult times.
3. Talk (support groups) and breathe (meditation).
4. Practice BLAH: no blame, animosity, or hard feelings.
5. Find the humor.

Friends and Family

1. Be honest.
2. Educate them.
3. Have some understanding that they have no idea what you are going through.
4. Don't allow unnecessary stress from friends or family members to bring you down.
5. Go CRAZY!

Job

1. Remember it is *just* a job. Your health is more important.
2. Educate management about your disease, but don't whine about it.
3. If you need to focus on a project, ask if you can go off to a quiet room to get it done.
4. If at all possible, don't take your work home with you.
5. If you are upset with coworkers, think before you speak.

Physical Aches and Pains

1. Take hot baths.
2. Exercise, stretching, and yoga can help.
3. Get massages.
4. Make a food diary. See if certain foods trigger the pain.
5. Take chromium picolinate (check with your MD beforehand). See "Chromium Picolinate and Joint Pain," http://www. livestrong.com/article/338915-chromium-picolinate-joint-pain/.

Lab Work

1. Find out from your MD exactly what they are testing; they are not always forthright with this information.
2. Research other tests you feel you might need.
3. If your MD does not agree to do testing that you think you need, go to an independent lab and get tested.
4. Research to see what is required prior to all testing (e.g., fasting, drinking water, etc.).
5. Require copies of all your lab work to come to you as well as the MD.

Spiritual

1. Read the word of God.
2. Be active in spiritual activities (for example, going to church). Help others within your community.
3. Pray.
4. Love others, including the ones who have wronged you. It took me awhile, but I've finally come around to loving those at The Pit. They were placed in my life for a reason.
5. Know and understand that God does not put more on you than you can handle.

Weight Loss

1. Eat as "clean" as possible: all organic and no processed foods.
2. Eat little or no gluten.
3. Be patient.
4. Exercise.
5. Work vigorously on digestive health by taking probiotics and a multivitamin. (I take 1-2 food-based organic multivitamins a day)
6. Try to eliminate diet drinks, caffeine, sugary drinks, and fruit juices. Drink plenty of water.
7. Drink noni juice.

Please note: These weight loss tips may sound extreme to you, but when you are without a fully functioning thyroid, they are a necessity. Not doing these things is literally like canoeing upstream without a paddle.

———

Your doctor should be made aware of any severe or troublesome symptoms associated with autoimmune and thyroid disease. I sought help for many of the issues below. When my doctor shrugged them off, I used MacGraver tricks to feel better. However, if any of my symptoms became too severe, I would *always* find another doctor to help me.

Insomnia: Try melatonin; see if your body can accept more than one.

Heart palpitations: Consume cayenne pepper. Check your iron and T3 levels, and exercise.

Diarrhea or constipation: Take fiber and eat balanced meals.

Muscle weakness, joint pain, or muscle wasting: Begin light or heavy weight training. Talk to your doctor and seek out a professional. You can also try physical therapy if you want insurance to pay for any weight-training tips.

Eye pain: Place a cool compress over your eyes for five to ten minutes and take ibuprofen as needed.

Depression, anxiety, and other mood changes: Pray, mediate, and destress as much as possible. Read, take long walks, do puzzles—whatever makes you happy.

Hair loss: I wear hair pieces. This can get expensive, but I cut other things out to afford them.

Memory issues: Take gingko biloba (check with your doctor beforehand). Play concentration games. A cool thing I started doing recently is tape-recording all MD instructions with my smart phone. I cannot trust my memory anymore, and I typically can't read their handwritten instructions.

Difficulty concentrating: When I am at work or at home and trying to concentrate on something, music (without words) or white noise helps me to focus.

Fatigue at work: Drink a large amount of water. When I find myself dozing off at work, I quickly drink three eight-ounce glasses of water. This trick will give you more energy than caffeine. Sometimes dehydration can cause extreme fatigue. Plus trips to the bathroom can wake you up. For more fatigue-fighting tips check out this link: http://thehealthyapron.com/2011/03/16/4-ways-to-increase-energy-and-fight-fatigue/

Heat intolerance/cold intolerance: Carry around extra clothing to put on or be prepared to take clothing off.

Restless legs: Get your iron and magnesium levels checked.

Hygiene: Carry around deodorant, Wisps (portable toothbrushes), and lotion in case you *forget* to use these items in the morning before you walk out of the house.

Vitamins, minerals, and hormones: I think most of us will agree that the medical community is reactive instead of proactive. Here are a few examples, my father collapsed a few years ago because his calcium levels were too low, and he had to be rushed to the hospital. My coworker told me about her friend who could not undergo a scheduled operation because after her blood results came back, it was determined that her potassium levels were too low. Her surgeon was afraid she would go into cardiac arrest on the operating table. It took over a month to boost her potassium levels before she could get the much-needed surgery. During a recent gynecological exam, my doctor decided to check some of my hormone levels (I had to beg him) and found that my progesterone was almost nonexistent in my body. And let us not forget the massive amount of people who are deficient in vitamin D. Many scientists believe these deficiencies could be the culprit in the upsurge of autoimmune diseases.

If the medical community actively tested our vitamin, mineral, and hormone levels yearly, I wonder if this could solve many of our health-care woes. I have worked in the health-care industry for more than ten years now, and I am also a seasoned patient, so I know that doctors and insurance companies will not enthusiastically sign off on lab work testing involving vitamins, minerals, or hormones. It seems that these tests are only run under the extremist of circumstances. Part of my MacGraver trickery is that I get my own lab testing done, independent of my doctor, if they deny my requests. If I feel like I may be deficient in an area, I will not hesitate to get that area tested.

Please look at this vitamin and mineral chart. Keep in mind your own nutritional dietary intake, as well as the deficiency information and see if perhaps you are lacking in one or more areas. Please do your own research on hormones. I did not include hormone data because the information for all of our human hormones is quite lengthy.

Good news! I have partnered with a company called Personal Labs. They are an independent lab with over 1,700 locations nationwide where you can get your own lab work done, bypassing your doctor. There are over four hundred tests offered. For my readers *only*, Personal Labs is offering a 5 percent discount, but you *must* use my code PLABSCTL (Personal Labs Crazy Thyroid Lady). Take control of your health!

VITAMINS

Vitamin	Good For	Toxicity	Deficiency	Soluble
A—Retinol	Vision, hair, skin	In general, acute toxicity occurs at doses of 25,000 IU/kg of body weight	Dry, hard eyeballs, Acne, Dry hair	Fat
B1—Thiamine	helps the body metabolize fats and proteins	Is Rare	Glaucoma Sensitivity to insect bites Furrowed tongue	Water
B2—Riboflavin	metabolism and for general good health	Primarily only with B2 Injections	Blurred vision Eczema, skin ulcers Dandruff Cracked lips & corners of the mouth	Water

B3—Niacin	controlling blood sugar, keeping healthy skin , and optimal functioning of the nervous and digestive systems	Could cause liver damage or flushing	Edema or tooth-marks on tongue Fingers white, numb, stiff, swellings (Raynaud's disease)	Water
B5—Pantothenic Acid	helps to reduce triglycerides and cholesterol levels	No reported side effects	Blurred vision White skin patches (vitiligo) Graying hair Beefy, enlarged tongue	Water
B6—Pyridoxine	Helps with mood	Can cause neurological problems and loss of sensation of arms and legs	Neuropathy, skin changes and confusion	Water
B7—Biotin	Healthy Skin and hair	No reported side effects	hair loss, cracking in the corners of the mouth, dry eyes and skin, tiredness, insomnia, depression and a flagging appetite	Water
B9—Folic Acid	Produce healthy red blood cells and prevent anemia	Low risk, but could cause seizures	Anemia	Water
B12—Cobalamins	Aids digestion, promotes brain health improves cholesterol levels	Rash	anemia, fatigue, weakness, constipation, loss of appetite, weight loss, depression, poor memory	Water

C— Ascorbic Acid	Growth and repair of tissues through the body	diarrhea, gas, or stomach upset	dry hair; gingivitis ; rough, dry, scaly skin; decreased wound-healing rate, easy bruising; and a decreased ability to ward off infection	Water
D— Calciferol	absorption and metabolism of calcium and phosphorous, immune system regulator	hypercalcaemia or hypercalcuria	Bone pain and tenderness, dental deformities	Fat
E— Tocopherol	protects cells, helps fight disease anti-aging properties	Blood thinning	Neurological disorders	Fat
K— Phylloquinone	Blood-clotting, bone health, anti-inflammatory brain functioning	Thrombosis	anemia, bruising, and bleeding of the gums or nose in both sexes, and heavy menstrual bleeding in women	Fat

Fat-soluble vitamins are stored in the fatty areas of the body. Since these vitamins are stored in fat, toxicity can occur if too much is taken. Water-soluble vitamins metabolize faster and typically flush out more quickly through urine. Toxicity for water-soluble vitamins is rare.

MINERALS

Mineral	Good for	Toxicity	Deficiency
Potassium	Nerve stimulation	hyperkalemia	Blood pressure problems
Chlorine	Chloride adjusts the alkali-acid equilibrium in the blood	hyperchloremia	body cramps
Sodium	Helps keep the right balance of fluid in the body	hypernatremia	Abnormal mental status Confusion; Decreased consciousness; Hallucinations
Calcium	Promotes, bone, teeth, muscle and nerve health	hypercalcaemia	affects bones and teeth and heart rhythm
Phosphorus	Aids digestive, nervous and the immune system	hyperphosphatemia	Weak bones or teeth, joint pain and stiffness, less energy and lack of appetite.
Magnesium	normal muscle and nerve function, keeps heart rhythm steady, supports a healthy immune system, and keeps bones strong	hypermagnesemia	dizziness, muscle cramps, muscle weakness and fatigue
Zinc	Plays a role in cell division, cell growth, wound healing, and the breakdown of carbohydrates.	anemia, liver and kidney damage	white spots on nails skin legions, acne, wasting of body tissues
Iron	Iron supplements are also used for increasing athletic performance, improving attention span in ADHD-affected children and healing canker sores and as an alternative treatment for Crohn's disease, infertility, depression and fatigue	Fever, chills and dizziness	anemia

Manganese	Help your body synthesize fatty acids and cholesterol	neurological symptoms consist of reduced response speed, irritability, mood changes, and compulsive behaviors	Ataxia, fainting, hearing loss, weak tendons and ligaments
Copper	Helps in the formation of red blood cells. It also helps in keeping the blood vessels, nerves, immune system, and bones healthy.	low blood pressure, vomiting jaundice	tiredness, fatigue, and light headedness
Iodine	needed for the normal metabolism of cells and thyroid function	Coughing, abdominal pain, diarrhea, delirium and fever.	goiter, mental retardation, weight gain
Selenium	help prevent cellular damage from free radicals	garlic odor on the breath, gastrointestinal disorders, hair loss, sloughing of nails, fatigue, irritability, and neurological damage	excessive fatigue, goiter, hypothyroidism
Molybdenum	needed for the normal metabolism of cells and thyroid function	Gout-like symptoms such as pain and swelling of joints	Headaches, night blindness, and an accelerated heart and respiratory rate.

The Final Scene

Wow, what a long, tumultuous journey! I persevered, with a small amount of help from various doctors, but the rest was up to me. Now I am gardening, playing with kids, and smiling at neighbors—not because I feel I have to in order to mask a damaged persona but because I have come out of the depths of sickness and despair. My annual trips to the ER with heart palpitations have ended. I don't spend the whole weekend in bed anymore. I am no longer depressed over my weight issues. I am not a ticking time bomb waiting to explode on someone because of emotions that have been amplified by my thyroid disease. I am happy! Truly happy! With cunning fortitude and prayer, I was able to fight my way back to functioning. I took control of and responsibility for my health. I did not get the help I thought I would after my diagnosis, so I had to empower myself. I wish there was a magic pill, a cure, but there isn't. At least not now.

So now I want to empower you to take ownership of your health. I know I have included a lot of information, but it takes a lot to tackle autoimmune thyroid disease. Health-care practitioners do not have all the answers; it is up to you to sit in the pilot's seat. Are you finding ways to keep your stress levels down? Are you eating nutritionally and exercising? Are you communicating with friends and family members in a positive way? And last, but certainly not least, are you working toward spiritual growth?

If you are not actively (and be honest with yourself) working to do all these things, then please don't wonder why you still feel crummy the majority of the time. Don't get me wrong; I still have bad days. But the bad days of old are far less common and not as severe as they used to be. I am a realist, and until there is a cure for my autoimmune disease, I may never be 100 percent. But I must continue to stay focused on my body and give it what it needs to stay well. It is a lot of work, but you and me are worth it.

And now we have come to the end. I want to take the time to thank each and every one of you for reading. Thanks so much for being a part my life and for putting up with my cathartic ramblings about The Pit, my difficult disease journey, and those added silly movie references. I would also like to thank the Academy, my husband for contributing to this book, the inept doctors I stumbled upon along the way, my son for his hard-working addition to the book, (just kidding he did most of the artwork). The Pit players, all of my editors, the MacGraver contributors, both my fathers in heaven (little *f* and big *F*), my mom and sister, all of my other family members, and, above all, I would like to thank Google!

The End

Roll the credits.

Resource Page

Thyroid Organizations

- **GRAVES' DISEASE AND THYROID FOUNDATION**
  P.O. Box 2793
  Rancho Santa Fe, CA 92067
  Toll Free National: 1-877-643-3123

- **AMERICAN THYROID ASSOCIATION**
  http://www.thyroid.org/

Thyroid Advocacy Groups

- **THYROID CHANGE**- An international, grass-roots initiative aiming to unite thyroid patients, physicians, websites, and organizations for improved thyroid disease management and treatment in the medical field.
  http://www.thyroidchange.org/

Thyroid Blogs

- **http://www.crazythyroidlady.blogspot.com/**

Thyroid internet videos

- **HOW THE BODY WORKS : THE THYROID GLAND**
  http://www.youtube.com/watch?v=7V0HB4cKIMw
- **Thyroid videos by Dr. Mary Hyman-Ultrawellness**

References

<http://webcache.googleusercontent.com/search?q=cache:5N5i2b Na5vgJ:www.ngdf.org/pages/6+thyroid+statistics+2010+-cancer& cd=1&hl=en&ct=clnk&gl=us>.

BIBLIOGRAPHY Benac, Eric. Ehow. 22 July 2011 <http://www. ehow.com/about_5373386_foods-contain-chlorine.html>.

Beckman, Mary. latimes.com. 24 September 2007. 25 May 2011 <http://articles.latimes.com/2007/sep/24/health/he-closer24>.

BIBLIOGRAPHY Bennett, A. (2010, August 24). *How to Cleanse Your Body Before Dieting.* Retrieved August 19, 2012, from LiveStrong: http://www.livestrong.com/article/107334-cleanse-body-before-dieting/

Cefik, Lisa. LiveStrong. 30 March 2011. 20 July 2011 <http:// www.livestrong.com/article/180231-what-is-vitamin-biotin-good-for/#ixzz1uPj3kjDL>

BIBLIOGRAPHY E. Blaurock-Busch, Ph.D. DrKaslow. 2011. <30>.

BIBLIOGRAPHY Ericka Grebel, PHD. Diabetes Forcast. March 2011. 25 August 2011 <http://forecast.diabetes.org/magazine/ diabetes-101/detecting-thyroid-disease>.

BIBLIOGRAPHY Fayed, Saad. About.com. 3 August 2011 <http://
mideastfood.about.com/od/tipsandtechniques/a/steaming.htm>.

Guttler, Dr. Richard. Thyroid.com. 2009. 10 June 2011 <http://
www.thyroid.com/patientinformation.html#socal>.

BIBLIOGRAPHY Jennifer Brett, N.D. Discovery Fit & Health.
21 July 2011 <http://health.howstuffworks.com/wellness/
food-nutrition/vitamin-supplements/benefits-of-vitamin-e.htm>.

BIBLIOGRAPHY Last, Walter. Defiency Symptoms. 22 July 2011
<http://www.health-science-spirit.com/deficiency.html>.

Mangano, Joseph J. Radiation.org. 12 May 2011 <http://www.
radiation.org/reading/pubs/091116Thyroidcancer.pdf>.

BIBLIOGRAPHY Mangano, Joseph. Thyroid Cancer Incident
Rate In Counties Closest to Nuclear Plants. 7 January 2012
<https://docs.google.com/viewer?a=v&q=cache:R4ChrF4hCVo
J:www.radiation.org/reading/pubs/091116Thyroidcancer.pdf+
&hl=en&gl=us&pid=bl&srcid=ADGEESi05qHxt3nErr9nKw
b_aKdNq0StcW2k_xhmjJ2vbXF-Gxt4pv5rc8xHMhotjlOinHLWk
uUwckN4WkPvhps5Yfyl_3UxyKDt5gK0HBZAySKeUCwjGM>.

Mayank, J. ehow.com. 1999. 20 July 2011 <http://www.ehow.
com/info_8102380_foods-away-energy.html>.

BIBLIOGRAPHY McRae, Shelly. 1999. 20 July 2011 <http://www.
ehow.com/how-does_4759213_junk-food-affect-health.html>.

Neil Solomon, M.D., Ph.D. "The Noni Solution." Solomon, Neil.
The Noni Solution. Orem: Direct Source Publishing, 2004. 272.

BIBLIOGRAPHY Unk. Reference Daily Intake. 12 August
2012. 22 September 2012 <http://en.wikipedia.org/wiki/
Reference_Daily_Intake>.

BIBLIOGRAPHY Unk. <u>Mecola.</u> 20 July 2011 <http://products. mercola.com/vitamine/>.

BIBLIOGRAPHY MsConnie. <u>LiveStrong.</u> 14 June 2011. 20 July 2011 <http://www.livestrong.com/article/286385-pyridoxine-toxicity/>.

Rodriguez, Diana. <u>everydayhealth.com.</u> 27 May 2009. 15 May 2011 <http://www.everydayhealth.com/thyroid-conditions/how-stress-affects-thyroid-problems.aspx>.

Shoman, Mary. <u>thyroid-info.com.</u> 1997. 17 December 2011 <http://www.thyroid-info.com/articles/tsh-fluctuating.htm>.

BIBLIOGRAPHY Shoman, Mary. <u>About.com.</u> 3 December 2003. 5 January 2012 <http://thyroid.about.com/cs/famouspeople/a/ devers.htm>.

Staff, Mayo Clinic. <u>mayoclinic.com.</u> 2011. 18 August 2011 <http://www.mayoclinic.com/health/graves-disease/DS00181/ DSECTION=symptoms>.

BIBLIOGRAPHY Steven D. Ehrlich, NMD. <u>University of Maryland Medical Center.</u> 1997. 20 July 2011 <http://www.umm. edu/altmed/articles/vitamin-b1-000333.htm>.

BIBLIOGRAPHY Terry, Sarah. <u>LiveStrong.</u> 14 August 2010. 19 July 2011 <http://www.livestrong.com/article/205376-what-is-vitamin-b5-good-for/>.

Thomas, Liana. <u>ehow.com.</u> 1999. 25 July 2011 <http://www. ehow.com/info_8094569_glutenfree-foods-energy.html>.

BIBLIOGRAPHY Tourney, Ann. <u>LiveStrong.</u> 1 February 2011. 31 July 2011 <http://www.livestrong.com/article/371139-molybdenum-deficiency-symptoms/#ixzz1uoEkZVjP>.

BIBLIOGRAPHY Tylee, Peter & Jenny. Healthy Vitamin Choice.
2005. 20 July 2011 <http://www.healthy-vitamin-choice.com/
vitamin-toxicity.html>.

BIBLIOGRAPHY Unk. 12step.org. 7 April 2012 <http://
www.12step.org/the-12-steps/step-3.html>.

BIBLIOGRAPHY Unk. Blurt it. 25 July 2011 <http://www.
blurtit.com/q425109.html>.

BIBLIOGRAPHY Unk. brainready.com. 20 July 2011 <http://
www.brainready.com/blog/thetop5brainhealthfoods.html>.

BIBLIOGRAPHY Unk. digestive.niddk.nih.gov. April 2008.
31 March 2011 <http://digestive.niddk.nih.gov/ddiseases/pubs/
yrdd/>.

Unk. Cancer.org. 17 September 2011 <http://www.cancer.
org/Treatment/TreatmentsandSideEffects/PhysicalSideEffects/
InfectionsinPeoplewithCancer/InfectionsinPeoplewithCancer/
infections-in-people-with-cancer-nutrition>.

—. CDC.gov. 10 September 2010. 20 July 2011 <http://www.cdc.
gov/mmwr/preview/mmwrhtml/mm5935a1.htm>.

BIBLIOGRAPHY Unk. CNR berkely. 22 July 2011 <http://cnr.
berkeley.edu/breakthroughs/break_feature2_fa07.php>.

Unk. commonsensefruit.com. 20 July 2011 <http://
commonsensehealth.com/Diet-and-Nutrition/Fruits_List_with_
Fruit_Nutritional_Value.shtml>.

BIBLIOGRAPHY Unk. Fit Sugar. 22 March 2007. 23 July
2011 <http://www.fitsugar.com/Vitamins-Water-Soluble-vs-Fat-
Soluble-181446>.

BIBLIOGRAPHY Unk. <u>Medline Plus.</u> 26 July 2011 <http://www. nlm.nih.gov/medlineplus/dietarysodium.html>.

BIBLIOGRAPHY Unk. <u>Medline Plus.</u> 20 July 2011 <http://www. nlm.nih.gov/medlineplus/ency/article/002416.htm>.

BIBLIOGRAPHY Unk. <u>Office of Dietary Supplements.</u> 22 July 2011 <http://ods.od.nih.gov/factsheets/Magnesium-HealthProfessional/>.

BIBLIOGRAPHY Unk. <u>totalhealthmagazine.com.</u> 21 July 2011 <http://www.totalhealthmagazine.com/Article/coveringalltheba. html>.

Unk. <u>Freedictionary.com.</u> 20 July 2011 <http://medical-dictionary. thefreedictionary.com/Fruit+Vegetable>.

BIBLIOGRAPHY Worden, Dr. Jen. <u>netdoctor.co.uk.</u> 20 July 2011 <http://www.netdoctor.co.uk/health_advice/facts/vitamins_which. htm>.

—. <u>Fruitsinfo.com.</u> 20 July 2011 <http://www.fruitsinfo.com/ simple_fruits.htm>.

—. <u>Graves' Disesae and Thyroid Foundation.</u> 2011. 7 September 2011 <http://www.gdatf.org/about/about-graves-disease/>.

unk. <u>iaff.org.</u> 20 July 2011 <http://www.iaff.org/ET/JobAid/EAP/ Poor_Nutrition.htm>.

—. <u>iloveindia.com.</u> 20 July 2011 <http://www.iloveindia.com/ nutrition/vegetable/types-of-vegetables.html>.

BIBLIOGRAPHY Unk. <u>Definitions of Doctor's Specialties.</u> 2012. 2 January 2012 <http://www.altabatessummit.org/physicians/ physician_specialty_definitions.html>.

BIBLIOGRAPHY Unk. Health Diaries. 4 March 2011. 23 July 2011 <http://www.healthdiaries.com/eatthis/6-health-benefits-of-vitamin-k.html>.

BIBLIOGRAPHY Unk. Health Suplements Nutrional Guide. 24 July 2011 <http://www.healthsupplementsnutritionalguide.com/Molybdenum.html#TOXICITY>.

BIBLIOGRAPHY Unk. Free dieting. 2001. 28 July 2011 <http://www.freedieting.com/food_guide_carbs.htm>.

BIBLIOGRAPHY Unk. Lupus Alliance. 12 June 2011 <http://www.lupusalliance.org/content.asp?id=557>.

BIBLIOGRAPHY Unk. medfasthealth. 1 August 2011 <http://www.medifasthealth.org/medifast-health/digestive-health.php>.

BIBLIOGRAPHY Unk. Medical News Today. 24 August 2009. 22 July 2011 <http://www.medicalnewstoday.com/articles/161618.php>.

BIBLIOGRAPHY Unk. NewsMax. 2011 March 2011. 21 July 2011 <http://www.newsmax.com/FastFeatures/health-benefits-of-vitamin/2011/03/01/id/387945>.

BIBLIOGRAPHY Unk. Office of Dietary Supplements. 21 July 2011 <http://ods.od.nih.gov/factsheets/Folate-HealthProfessional/>.

BIBLIOGRAPHY Unk. projectavalon.net. 1 August 2011 <http://projectavalon.net/forum/archive/index.php/t-10577.html>.

BIBLIOGRAPHY Unk. Pub Med Health. 3 August 2010. 24 July 2011 <http://www.ncbi.nlm.nih.gov/pubmedhealth/PMH0001384/#adam_000344.disease.symptoms>.

BIBLIOGRAPHY Unk. Scientific American. 27 July 2011 <http://www.scientificamerican.com/article.cfm?id=vitamin-d-and-autism>.

BIBLIOGRAPHY Unk. Thesaurus. <http://thesaurus.com/>.

BIBLIOGRAPHY Unk. University of Maryland Medical Center. 22 July 2011 <http://www.umm.edu/altmed/articles/vitamin-c-000339.htm>.

BIBLIOGRAPHY Unk. WebMD. 27 July 2011 <http://women.webmd.com/features/life-with-autoimmune-disease?page=2>.

Unk. WebMD. 27 July 2011. 5 August 2011 <http://www.webmd.com/cancer/tc/thyroid-cancer-symptoms>.

BIBLIOGRAPHY Unk. Wikipedia. 21 July 2011 <http://en.wikipedia.org/wiki/Dietary_mineral>.

BIBLIOGRAPHY Unk. Wikipedia. 25 July 2011 <http://en.wikipedia.org/wiki/Immunology>.

BIBLIOGRAPHY Unk. Wikipedia. 24 July 2011 <http://en.wikipedia.org/wiki/Retinol#Immune_system>.

BIBLIOGRAPHY Unk. Wikipedia. 27 July 2011 <http://en.wikipedia.org/wiki/Magnesium_deficiency_(medicine)>.

BIBLIOGRAPHY Unk. Wikipedia. 20 July 2011 <http://en.wikipedia.org/wiki/Thiamine>.

BIBLIOGRAPHY Unk. Wikipedia. 20 July 2011 <http://en.wikipedia.org/wiki/Pantothenic_acid>.

BIBLIOGRAPHY Unk. Wikipedia. 20 July 2011 <http://en.wikipedia.org/wiki/Phosphorus_deficiency>.

BIBLIOGRAPHY Unk. <u>Wikipedia.</u> 20 July 2011 <http://en.wikipedia.org/wiki/Pyridoxine>.

BIBLIOGRAPHY Unk. <u>Wikipedia.</u> 20 July 2011 <http://en.wikipedia.org/wiki/Pyridoxine_deficiency>.

BIBLIOGRAPHY Unk. 20 July 2011 <http://en.wikipedia.org/wiki/Vitamin_A#Toxicity>.

BIBLIOGRAPHY Unk. <u>Wikipedia.</u> 20 July 2011 <http://en.wikipedia.org/wiki/Tocopherol>.

BIBLIOGRAPHY Unk. <u>Wikipedia.</u> 23 July 2011 <http://en.wikipedia.org/wiki/Selenium#Toxicity>.

BIBLIOGRAPHY Unk. <u>Wikepedia.</u> 20 July 2011 <http://en.wikipedia.org/wiki/Vitamin>.

BIBLIOGRAPHY Unk. <u>Wiki Answers.</u> 9 September 2011 <http://wiki.answers.com/Q/What_does_'organic'_mean>.

BIBLIOGRAPHY Unk. <u>Weird Asia News.</u> 2006. 12 May 2012 <http://www.weirdasianews.com/2011/05/23/chinese-man-afflicted-orange-peel-hands-feet/>.

BIBLIOGRAPHY Unk. <u>What is a Serving Size.</u> 21 July 2011 <http://www.fns.usda.gov/tn/healthy/portions_kit/serving_size.pdf>.

BIBLIOGRAPHY Unk. <u>Womens Health.</u> 18 May 2010. 12 September 2011 <http://www.womenshealth.gov/publications/our-publications/fact-sheet/graves-disease.cfm>.

BIBLIOGRAPHY Unk. <u>The World's Healthiest Foods.</u> 27 July 2011 <http://www.whfoods.com/genpage.php?tname=nutrient&dbid=77>.

BIBLIOGRAPHY Unk. World's Healthiest Foods. 24 July 2011
<http://whfoods.org/genpage.php?tname=dailytip&dbid=3>.

Unk. Bestinseason.ie. 20 July 2011 <http://www.bestinseason.ie/
whats-in-season/>.

—. CDC.gov. 20 July 2011 <http://www.fruitsandveggiesmatter.
gov/benefits/>.

—. Encyclopedia. 7 August 2011 <www.encyclopedia.com/topic/
Autoimmune_diseases.aspx+thyroid+autoimmune+disease+facts+st
atistics+-cANCER&cd=21&hl=en&ct=clnk&gl=us>.

—. EveryNutrient.com. 24 November 2011 <http://www.
everynutrient.com/healthbenefitsofgarlic.html>.

www.ingramcontent.com/pod-product-compliance
Lightning Source LLC
Chambersburg PA
CBHW020437290526
45785CB00002B/899